cure and recognize aquarium fish diseases

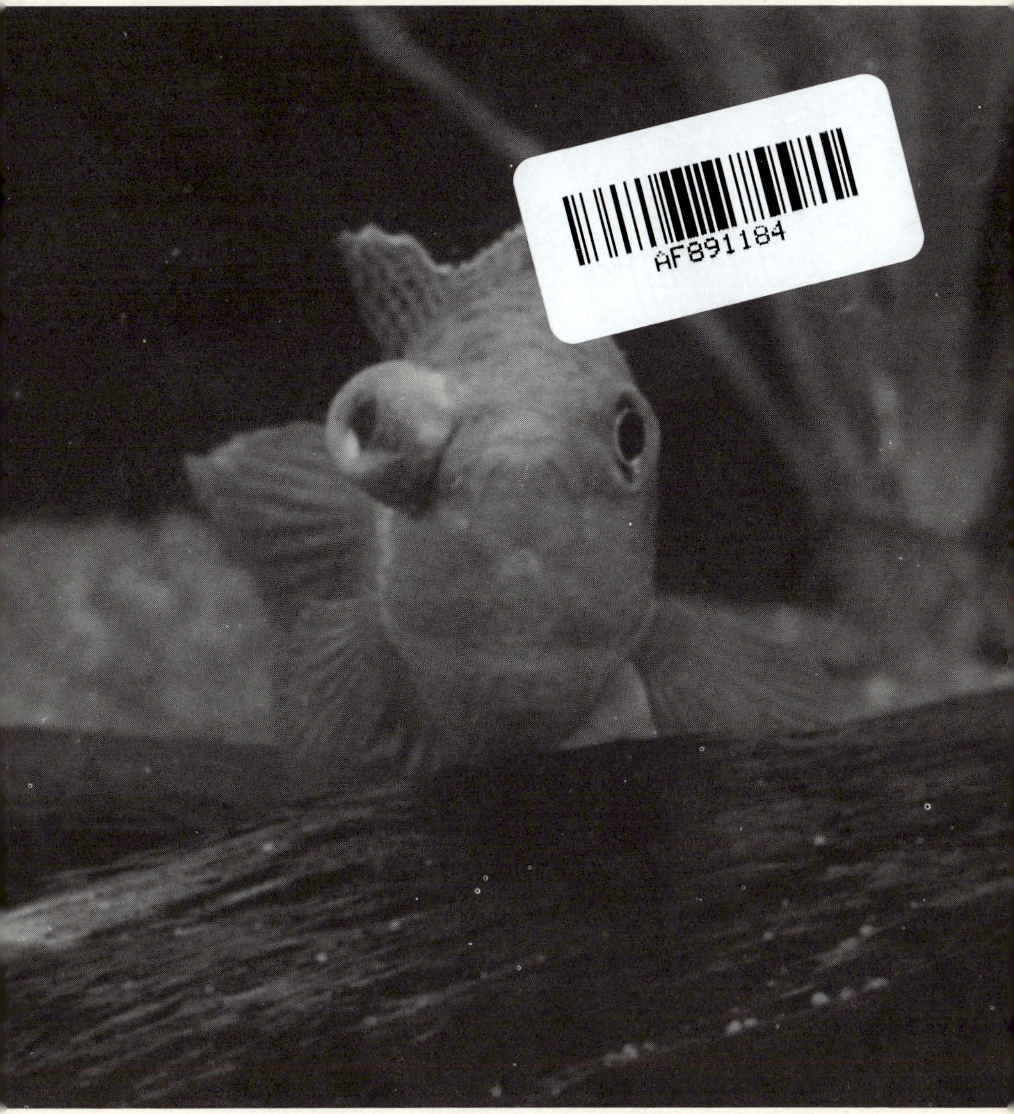

by dr. gottfried schubert
translated by christa ahrens

Line drawings are from Dr. Schubert's *Krankheiten der Fische*, published by Franckh'sche Verlagshandlung, W. Keller & Co., Stuttgart.

ISBN 0-87666-033-2

Distributed in the U.S.A. by T.F.H. Publications, Inc., 211 West Sylvania Avenue, P.O. Box 27, Neptune City, N.J. 07753; in England by T.F.H. (Gt. Britain) Ltd., 13 Nutley Lane, Reigate, Surrey; in Canada to the book store and library trade by Clarke, Irwin & Company, Clarwin House, 791 St. Clair Avenue West, Toronto 10, Ontario; in Canada to the pet trade by Rolf C. Hagen Ltd., 3225 Sartelon Street, Montreal 382, Quebec; in Southeast Asia by Y.W. Ong, 9 Lorong 36 Geylang, Singapore 14; in Australia and the south Pacific by Pet Imports Pty. Ltd., P.O. Box 149, Brookvale 2100, N.S.W., Australia. Published by T.F.H. Publications Inc. Ltd., The British Crown Colony of Hong Kong.

CONTENTS

Foreword

Over a decade has elapsed since the first edition of *Diseases of Fishes* was published in Germany. Since then, new diseases have cropped up in our aquaria, our knowledge has increased and new practical experience has been gained. For these reasons, the present 5th edition has been completely revised.

Even more than before, I have endeavored to adapt the book to the practical needs of tropical fish keeping. Only those diseases which actually do occur in ornamental tropical fishes are dealt with. In the diagnostic sections, the aim has been to enable the interested layman, once he has gained the basic experience, to make a reliable diagnosis of these diseases. Here I have been able to benefit from the numerous suggestions that hobbyists have submitted to me.

In the chapter on therapeutic agents I have deliberately confined myself to a small number of reliable, effective drugs. However, in view of the constant rapid progress that is being achieved in this particular field, I would urge the reader to keep up to date with the help of aquarium magazines. It would be impossible, in a book of this scope, to deal with the immense profusion of therapeutic agents that are available on the market. It is up to the individual aquarist to gain the necessary critical experience at selecting and using the proper drugs.

Stuttgart GOTTFRIED SCHUBERT

Required instruments

Capture bells: The use of a net when catching diseased fish in a tank should be avoided whenever possible since any deposits on the skin likely to be of interest to us might all too easily be rubbed off. The best thing to do is to purchase one large and one small capture bell. These are similar to funnels with long stems and are simply placed over the fish. The small one is used for close scrutiny of the patients, the large one for catching. Inside its tube small fish can be easily examined through a magnifying glass, as they cannot turn around in it.

Net: For catching large cichlids and similar fishes, a net is imperative. It is also needed to drive the fish into the glass capture bell.

Pipette: To take parasites from inside the gill cavity we need a pipette with a rubber bulb. Ideally, the end should be thin and smoothed off in a Bunsen flame.

Dissecting pan: We will frequently find it necessary to dissect fish, and for this we need a dissecting pan. This can easily be made at home by using a shallow baking pan which is at least $1\frac{1}{2}$ times the length and 2 times the width of our biggest fish and has a depth of 5–7 cm (2–3 inches). Into this we pour some wax to form a layer of 1.5–2 cm ($\frac{5}{8}$–$\frac{7}{8}$ inch) thickness. Sheet zinc is best suited for the dish, but any material that can be heated to above the melting point of the wax will do. For the lining we use paraffin wax (old candle-ends, etc.), mixed with 5 to 10% ceresine or bees' wax to soften it a little. The fish is placed in this dish and fastened with pins so that both our hands remain free for dissecting and we can, if necessary, dissect under water. When, in time, the wax begins to look too perforated and worn, place it in a low temperature oven until it becomes smooth again.

Scissors: To open up the bigger fishes, a strong pair of scissors is required, preferably with one blade having a blunt and the other a sharp end. A second pair of scissors—finer, with two pointed ends—is used for the internal organs and the dissection of small fishes.

Forceps: We require one large, blunt pair and one or two small pairs of forceps, the latter with sharp points. Each of them needs to have a good grip at the tips, or else it would be impossible to keep hold of the slippery piece of fish skin.

Scalpel: A sharp-pointed scalpel with a metal handle frequently proves useful but is not absolutely essential.

Dissection needles: These are fine needles (sharp, blunt or lancet-like) with a handle. They are used for delicate probing and for separating and holding down tissues and organs. If you wish to purchase them, you are advised to choose holders with replaceable needles. Equally good are insect or hat pins which can be inserted into suitable wooden dowels. It is often useful to flatten the tip of one needle and file down an edge as a micro-scalpel.

Magnifying glasses: It is essential to have two magnifying glasses: a weaker one which magnifies approximately 3 times, and a more powerful one which magnifies approximately 10–12 times. The weak one enables us to carry out examinations from a distance (approximately 8 cm ($3\frac{1}{4}$ inches)) of an animal inside the capture bell, for instance. The more powerful magnifying glass with a working distance of about 2 cm ($\frac{7}{8}$ inch) can only be used on a dead animal. Multi-lens magnifying glasses designed to give more than one magnification (3 times, 6 times and 9 times, for instance, depending on whether the first lens is used alone, or only the second lens or the two of them together) are often quite practical, but they have the disadvantage that the visual field, as far as the weak lens is concerned, is smaller than it is in a magnifying glass designed solely for this magnification.

Microscope: Certain investigations are impossible to carry out without a microscope. The instrument does not have to be an expensive one; a simple microscope with magnifications within the range of 30 to 500 times is sufficient. Aquarium societies could help their members by acquiring this type of equipment.

Microscope slides: These are rectangular pieces of thin glass (standard size 76 × 26 mm (about 3 × 1 inches)) on which the material is put for examination through the microscope.

Cover slips: These are very thin glass plates or circles, for our purposes usually measuring about 18 × 18 mm ($\frac{3}{4}$ inch) and having a thickness of approximately 0.17 mm, that are used to cover the samples placed on the microscope slides. Microscope slides and cover slips are useful aids not only for work at the microscope, but also for examining translucent objects with the magnifying glass.

Graduated pipettes: These are required when we want to measure small quantities of therapeutic agents in solution. Sufficient for our purposes are one 2 ml pipette subdivided into units of 1/100 ml and one 10 ml pipette subdivided into units of 1/10 ml (1 ml = 1 cm^3 = 1 ccm (about a thousandth of a quart)). The solution is siphoned off with the mouth (CAUTION! Make sure none of the fluid gets into your mouth!), and the top opening of the pipette is then closed with the finger. By carefully relaxing the pressure of the finger, the fluid is allowed to escape drop by drop. The pipettes have been graduated in such a way that a given quantity is correct when no more fluid escapes and the tube is empty except for a few drops remaining inside the tapered end. Do not blow out! The pipettes have to be rinsed thoroughly after every use. It is a good idea to have a separate pipette for each solution.

Burette: Larger volumes of fluid are measured with burettes, which are graduated upright tubes made of glass or plastic. A burette with a capacity of 100 ml ($\frac{1}{5}$ pint) is sufficient. For quantities exceeding this we use an ordinary kitchen measuring pitcher.

Examination of a fish

For each individual investigated, we keep a file. Here is an example of such a record:

Investigation No.: Date:

Species: Sex: Age:

Origin: alive; killed; has been dead for:

Tank:

History:

Examination:

Diagnosis: Treatment:

Result:

In time, the collection of such data will enable us to draw such valuable conclusions as, for example, that we should no longer purchase our stock at breeder X or Y as his tanks are infected, or that a disease breaks out whenever our fish have been given foods from certain waters. Give as detailed an account as possible. Under "History" put down everything known about a particular fish and what has been observed so far. When carrying out the examination, methodically go through all the points listed in the diagnosis table and record what strikes one as abnormal.

In the table you will find that, under the various signs, reference has been made to the diseases that may be responsible for them. Simply check the discussion of the disease or condition in the text and determine whether it might be the disease your animals are

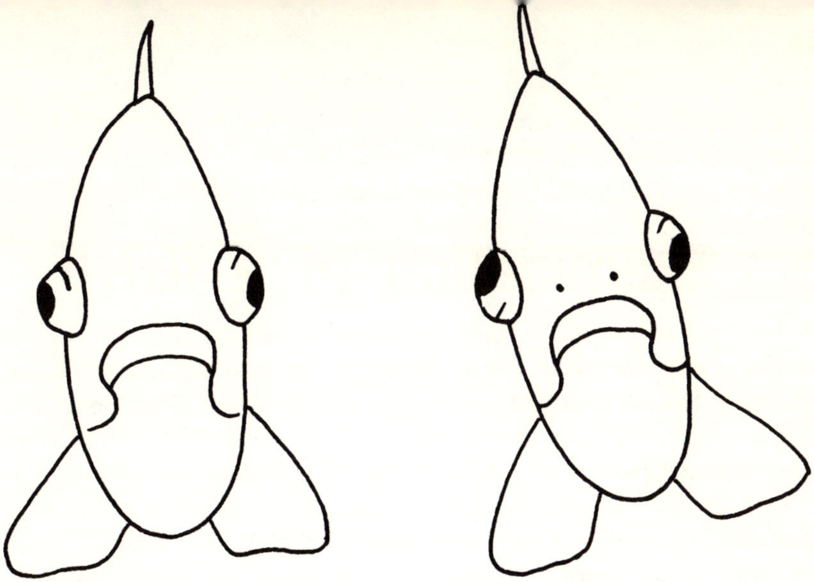

The ocular reflex. Notice that an off-balance fish tries to keep its gaze horizontal.

suffering from. Where the signs admit of several possibilities, the description of these diseases should make it quite easy to recognize which of them is present in any particular case. After the description of the disease, methods of treatment are mentioned.

The first part of the table deals with signs that can be observed in the living fish. Apart from supplying the first clues as to the nature of the disease, these signs tell us which organs we need to examine with particular thoroughness.

Wherever possible, a sample of newly deposited excreta is removed from the aquarium with a pipette and placed on a microscope slide to be examined under the microscope.

The fish has to be caught with great care and without being chased. Using the table as a step-by-step guide, first of all examine everything that can be examined while the fish is still swimming in the bell. For each subsequent check the fish has to be taken out of the water for a short period.

Begin by testing the ocular reflex. A healthy fish always attempts to maintain its gaze in a horizontal direction. If the fish is turned to the left or right, it will adjust its gaze accordingly. When this reflex is absent it is important, during subsequent investigations, to take particularly careful note of the condition of the brain.

Larger fishes complicate the examination by the resistance they offer. Anyone who is jabbed by the spines in the dorsal fin of certain fishes is easily induced to drop the fish. In such cases it is preferable to anaesthetize the fish prior to examination. *Important:* Poisonous fishes (lionfish, stonefish, etc.) should never be examined by the hobbyist, neither with an anaesthetic nor without.

In the case of skin turbidity or deposits on the skin, prepare a skin smear. The smear is taken with a blunt object (the blunt side of the scalpel or with a blunt spatula) which, in the direction of the tail, is lightly scraped over the conspicuous areas. The mucus that has been scraped off is put on a microscope slide, a little water is stirred in and the preparation covered with a cover slip. With a powerful magnifying glass or, preferably, with the microscope, check the scraping for parasites. India ink may be added to the water at a ratio of 1:10 to show the parasites as light objects against the dark background.

To examine the gills, a small pipette, smoothed off at the bottom and equipped with a rubber bulb, is inserted underneath the operculum; a little water is sprayed into the gill cavity and sucked back into the pipette immediately. The contents of the pipette are transferred onto a microscope slide, covered with a cover slip and examined under the microscope. If parasites are present on the gills in large numbers, they are certain to be found in this way without the fish having to be sacrificed. Isolated parasites may escape detection when this method is used, but they have little influence on the condition of the fish.

This examination should only be carried out on an anaesthetized fish; otherwise the animal might struggle so violently that its gills could be badly damaged and it could sustain fatal wounds.

If the observations made so far do not enable us to come to any definite conclusion, further investigations need to be carried out, and for these the fish has to be killed. With the possible exception of very valuable single specimens, this should really always be done since a disease rarely affects one fish only, but rather endangers all the inhabitants of the tank. The decision to sacrifice one fish while in return being given the chance to save all the others can hardly be a difficult one.

Where an examination of the blood can be dispensed with (and within the scope of our possibilities and purpose such an examination is of value only with regard to a few fishes such as goldfish, carp, Crucian carp, minnows, stickleback and African cichlids) the quickest and surest way of killing the fish is to cut deeply through the spine with scissors immediately behind the head. Other possible methods include immersion of the fish in a fairly strong anaesthetic solution where they will die in deep narcosis, or conduction of an electric current into the water. Both methods have disadvantages. Any parasites that may be attached are likely to leave the fish once it is unconscious and hence escape our notice. To meddle with power currents and water is extremely dangerous and I strongly advise against it. The cut through the spinal cord remains the quickest and most considerate method of sacrifice. Anyone who regards this method as too bloody should bear in mind that what matters in this particular circumstance is that the fish is being killed as quickly and painlessly as possible, not that one's own 'nerves' are being spared.

If we wish to examine the blood, the fish is made deeply unconscious with an anaesthetic or killed by an electric current. We then dry the posterior end of the animal thoroughly and with one cut separate the tail at the peduncle from the body. The blood dripping down is caught on a microscope slide and diluted with a 0.9% solution of sodium chloride (9 g of kitchen salt to 1 liter (about a quart) of water). Under the microscope check the blood for parasites by using a low-power (50 times) objective to start with and then more powerful (up to 300 times) objectives.

From the dead fish obtain another skin smear. This time scrape a bit more firmly and use the edge of a microscope slide. Explore particularly the bases of the dorsal and caudal fins, the axillae of the pectoral fins and the area along the lateral line. We also look at a piece of fin under the microscope at low and medium magnification. Next remove the gill operculum. From a smaller fish entire gill arches, and from a larger fish several gill filaments, are placed on an object slide and observed through a magnifying glass or the microscope. Afterwards the fish is cut open.

The most convenient way of doing this is to put the fish in the dissecting pan and hold it in place with pins. Carefully introduce one blade of the scissors close to the anus and cut along the medial line of the abdomen until reaching the gill region. The second incision is made in a semi-circle leading from the anus through the lateral surface of the body and terminating just above the operculum. It is important not to cut too deeply in order to avoid damaging any of the internal organs. The triangular strip of abdominal wall now free on two sides is lifted up in the anal region, and with the handle of the scalpel or a blunt pair of forceps any internal organs adhering to it are pushed back. Then we connect Incisions 1 and 2 by means of Incision 3. Remove the resulting strip of skin with another cut parallel to the operculum. The flap thus removed should be saved as the kidneys may frequently be attached to it. Note whether the abdominal cavity is filled with fluid (ascites). If the incisions have caused a lot of bleeding, which means we have been making mistakes, rinse the fish under running water.

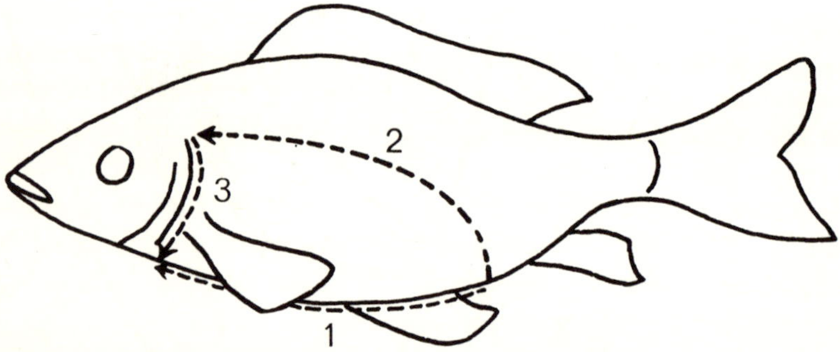

The use of three connected incisions allows the easy removal of musculature without disturbing the internal organs.

The various organs are now spread out a little. Often they are easier to spread out when the dissecting pan has been filled with water. Hidden between the loops of the intestine lies the spleen, easily recognized by its deep red color. It does not become visible until the intestine has been spread out.

Using the diagnosis table as a guide, examine the organs with the naked eye and the magnifying glass. Where necessary, make macerated and squash preparations by teasing the fragments of an

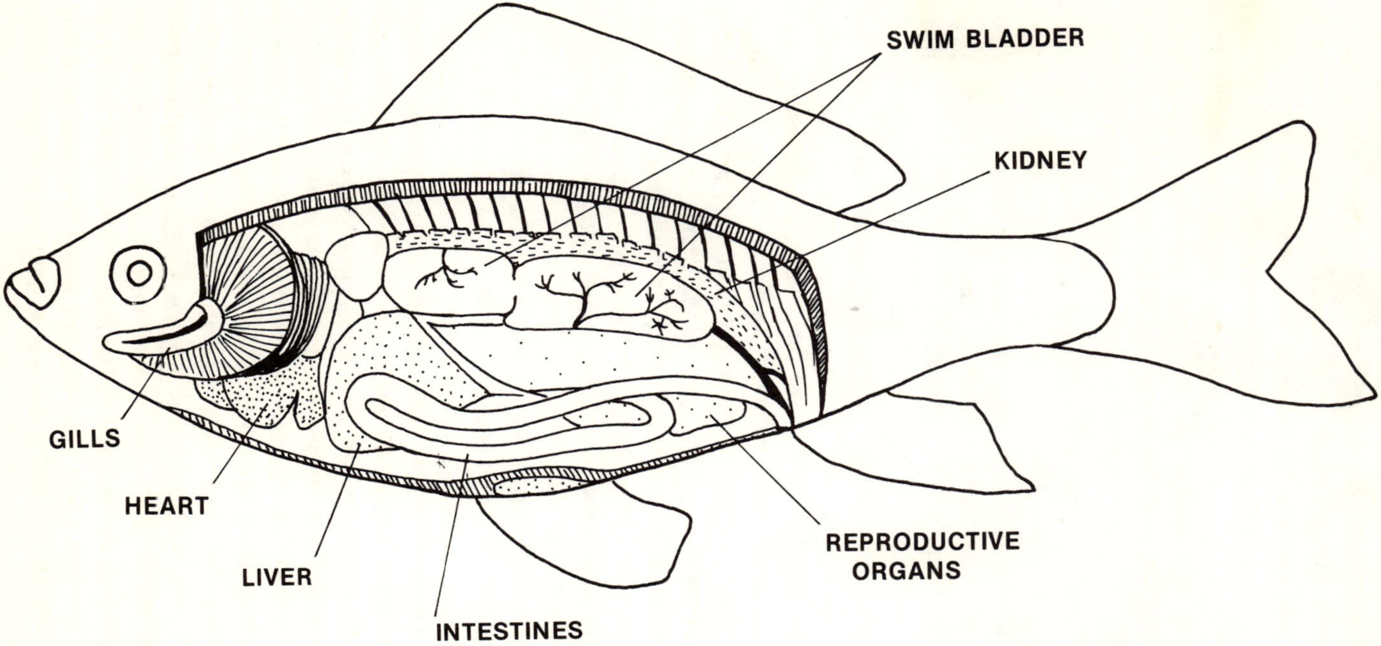

Generalized internal anatomy of a fish. The relative size and position of the organs vary somewhat in different groups of fishes.

organ with two needles or adding a little water and squeezing the tissue between microscope slide and cover slip. Cover slips break easily, so cover your thumb with a heavy paper towel before applying *even* pressure. The preparations are examined under the microscope or with a powerful magnifying glass.

Squash preparations do not give any information about the structure of the organs, since the natural architecture has been destroyed, but the presence of parasites is usually very obvious. The liver preparation, apart from containing liver cells and red blood corpuscles, will frequently reveal yellow granules which consist of hemosiderin. In small quantities these are present in almost every liver, but their occurrence in quantity indicates that something is wrong. If we, therefore, observe a large number of yellow granules, we have to carry out a particularly thorough check for parasites. In squash preparations of the kidney, the renal tubes should still be discernible, provided we did not put too much pressure on the cover slip, and any parasites that may be present will show up very clearly against them. When looking at the muscle preparation, the muscle fibers and often their cross striations as well can be seen. Parasites embedded in the muscles are considerably less transparent than their environment.

The intestine is opened by making a longitudinal incision. Prepare a smear from its contents and investigate it under the microscope. Finally, open up the skull. This is done by cutting from the left and right nasal openings towards the back (always holding the scissors flat) and connecting the two incisions at the front by cutting across between the nostrils. When this strip of tissue is lifted the brain is exposed. From this organ, too, a squash preparation is made. It is not necessary, for our purposes, to open up the cranium unless absence of ocular reflex or abnormal movement causes us to suspect that the brain has been damaged.

Diagnosis of Fish Diseases

Table I: Examination of the living fish

	Sign	*Possible diagnosis*
	Signs become apparent within a short period (a few hours to 1 day), when all or most of the animals die. Some species not affected, but of those which are, all animals suffer from the disease	Poisoning caused by unsuitable water. Check pH, carbon dioxide content, oxygen content, copper, zinc, phenols. Disturbances connected with feeding.
Behavior	The fish jump, move jerkingly	Acidosis, alkalosis. Poisoning caused by plant-protective chemicals.
	Gasping for air, irregular breathing, fish hanging at the surface	Lack of oxygen, ammonia poisoning, nitrite poisoning. Examine the gills.
	Respiratory rate abnormally fast, opercula moving faster than usual; apart from this behavior more or less normal	Gill parasites; examine the gills.
	Immediately after the onset of signs, the animals stand motionless and die	Carbon dioxide poisoning.
	Abnormal swimming position	*Cryptobia;* examine brain and air bladder as per Table II.

	Sign	*Possible diagnosis*
	Animals listless and in extreme cases can be caught with the hand	*Cryptobia*. Observed in many diseases at an advanced stage.
Skeleton and body form	Emaciation	Occurs in a number of diseases. Check above all for *Ichthyosporidium*, piscine tuberculosis.
	Curvature of the spine	*Camallanus*, sporozoan infection, piscine tuberculosis. In fry: developmental or congenital defects; destroy these animals.
	Distension	*Ichthyosporidium*, piscine tuberculosis, abdominal dropsy. Also occurring in other diseases.
	Neck tumor, perhaps with inability to close the mouth	Thyroid tumor, other tumors.
	Exophthalmos (= staring eyes)	Non-specific; check above all for fish tuberculosis, *Ichthyosporidium*, sparganosis (under Cestodes), metacercarial diseases, various bacterial diseases.
	When the fish is motionless, reddish worms can be seen to protrude from its anus, particularly in live-bearers	*Camallanus*.
Color	Colors always pale	Various diseases, unsuitable conditions (too bright, no hiding places, water too soft or too hard, pH, etc.).

	Sign	Possible diagnosis
	Dark to black coloration, partial or complete	*Ichthyosporidium, Hexamita,* melanosarcoma, damage of the nervous system due to injury or parasites.
	Whitish areas under the skin	*Plistophora* or other sporozoans, "false neon tetra disease."
	White mouth region, especially in live-bearers (with the exception of the guppy)	Columnaris disease.
Body surface	Egg sacs hanging from fish's body in clusters	*Lernaea* and related species.
	Raised scales	Bacterial infections, columnaris disease, dietary disorders. Examine skin smear.
	Crustaceans on the skin, particularly on the dorsal fin	*Argulus.*
	Fine to coarse deposits on the skin	Skin parasites. Examine skin smear.
	Up to 1 mm long, semolina-like deposits on the skin	In freshwater: *Ichthyophthirius.* In salt-water: *Cryptocaryon,* sporozoans. Examine skin smear.
	White, cottonwool-like deposits on the skin	Saprolegniacea. Check skin smear.
	Similar but finer threads, often in isolated areas	Columnaris disease, *Spironucleus.* Examine skin smear.
	Skin as if corroded, milky turbidity, inflammation, excessive mucus	Acidosis, alkalosis, *Costia,* especially in fishes with long fins. Examine skin smear.

	Sign	*Possible diagnosis*
	Spherical protrusions, up to 2 mm, firm to the touch, observed particularly on the fins, looking like spawn that has adhered to the skin; transparent	*Lymphocystis.*
	Small blisters under the skin; large fishes rustle when taken out of the water	Gas bubble disease.
	Reddish to black nodules	Metacercariae.
	Reddish inflamed areas, later turning grayish-white	*Argulus.*
	Circular inflamed areas	Leeches.
	White nodules in the skin, particularly on the fins; non-transparent	Sporozoans. Scrape or cut out nodules, make squash preparations and examine with the microscope.
	Unevenly distributed wounds	Mechanical injuries.
	Fin injuries, fraying of the fins, fins coming away	Bacterial fin rot, Saprolegniacea, columnaris disease, "false neon tetra disease," fish tuberculosis, *Ichthyosporidium.*
Skin smear	Small worms	Monogenea.
	Bean-shaped, small, highly motile flagellates	*Costia.*
	Circular ciliates, with ring of hooks, rotary motion	*Trichodina.*

	Sign	*Possible diagnosis*
	Blunt oval to heart-shaped ciliates, motile	*Chilodonella.*
	Small attached ciliates with stalk, only the ring of cilia being motile	*Glossatella.*
	Large round ciliates without ring of hooklets, rotary motion	In freshwater: *Ichthyophthirius.* In sea-water: *Cryptocaryon.*
	Casket-shaped protozoan, yellowish to brownish, nucleus lighter but usually indistinct, non-motile	*Oodinium.*
	Mycotic threads	Saprolegniacea.
	Very fine filaments, leave the smear and attach them-themselves to the cover-slip	Columnaris disease.
Gills (examination of material removed with a pipette)	All the signs listed under skin smear	
	Worms' eggs with or without adhesive threads	Monogenea.
	Hat-shaped worms' eggs	*Sanguinicola.*
Feces	Numerous highly motile flagellates	*Spironucleus.*
	Worms' eggs with button-like ends	*Capillaria.*
	Other worms' eggs	Various Digenea, nematodes, cestodes.

Sign	Possible diagnosis
Small, thin, colorless larvae of worms	*Camallanus.*
Long, oval ciliates, terminating in a sharp point at one end	Discus parasite.

Table II: Examination of the sacrificed fish

	Sign	*Possible diagnosis*
Blood	Flagellates, very motile, about the length of a blood-cell	*Cryptobia, Trypanosoma.*
Skin smear	As per Table I	
Gills	As per Table I	
	In addition, in squash preparations nodules of varying length release large numbers of spores.	Sporozoans.
	Brown deposits	Acidosis.
	Pale	Alkalosis.
	Crustaceans with clasping hooks	Ergasilidae.
	Inside the gills, granules arranged in rows, highly refractile	Indicating a metabolic disturbance, kidney damage, common in *Spironucleus* infection or in fish kept in unsuitable water.

	Sign	*Possible diagnosis*
Abdominal cavity	Filled with fluid	"Abdominal dropsy," metabolic disturbance.
	Cysts containing the larvae of worms	
	(a) Larvae with a proboscis armed with rings of hooklets	*Acanthocephalus.*
	(b) Larvae with a flat ring of hooks and/or suckers, or without either, in which case the shape of the larva is irregular; cyst frequently containing highly refractile bodies	Sparganosis, cestodes.
	(c) Larvae with suckers, isolated larva showing forked intestine	Digenea.
	(d) Larvae thin and worm-shaped, pointed at both ends, usually coiled like a spiral	Nematodes.
	Internal organs grown together, sometimes inflamed	Abdominal dropsy, bacterial infections.
	Liver green in places	Biliary stasis, *Hexamita*, other diseases, dietary disturbances.
	Liver yellowish or reddish-black instead of vermilion	Pathologic changes in the liver occur in many diseases.
Squash preparations of internal organs	Flagellates inside the gall bladder	*Hexamita*
	Flagellates in the intestine, liver, kidney and other organs	*Spironucleus.*

	Sign	Possible diagnosis
	Nodules with numerous spherical spores	Sporozoans.
	Cysts that vary in size, usually with dark to black pigment bodies	*Ichthyosporidium*, piscine tuberculosis.
	Larvae of worms—see under Abdominal cavity	
	Liver containing numerous fat globules	Fatty degeneration—diet not varied enough, vitamin deficiency. (In some species of fish the presence of fat in the liver is normal.)
	Hat-shaped worms' eggs, found particularly in the liver and kidney	*Sanguinicola.*
Intestine and intestinal contents	Sac-shaped worms attached to intestinal wall by spiny proboscis	Acanthocephala.
	Thread-like worms, female found to contain eggs or larvae	Nematodes.
	Thread-like worms, red, brown head capsule, found in the rectum	*Camallanus.*
	Worms with head-like bulge at one end	*Caryophyllaeus.*
	Worms with sucking grooves (bothria) or acetabuli, only at the front end	Cestodes.

	Sign	*Possible diagnosis*
	Worms with one acetabulum at the front end and another nearer the posterior end	Digenea.
	Spherical to casket-shaped protozoan, non-motile	*Oodinium.*
Squash preparations of the musclature	Cysts containing larvae of worms (see Abdominal cavity)	
	Cysts containing numerous bodies	*Plistophora.*
Eye, squash preparations of the tissues surrounding the eye	Cysts of varying size, usually containing dark brown to black pigment granules	*Ichthyosporidium,* piscine tuberculosis.
	Cysts containing the larvae of worms (see Abdominal cavity)	
	Gaseous blisters in the eye	Bacterial infection.
Squash preparation of the brain	Cysts with numerous internal bodies	Sporozoans.
	Cysts of varying size, usually with dark, brown to black pigment granules	*Ichthyosporidium,* piscine tuberculosis.

The Diseases

A.—Diseases caused by parasites

MANY-CELLED ORGANISMS (METAZOA)

Organisms composed of many cells.

Lower Crustacea (Entomostraca)

A few species among the relatives of *Cyclops* and *Daphnia*, which are so popular and valuable as fish foods, constitute a potential danger to our fishes.

CARP LICE *(Argulus)*

Etiology: The larvae of carp lice (several species) as well as the adult animals can injure the fish skin with stinging mouthparts equipped with a poison gland. Owing to the perforations and the perpetually moving legs of this crustacean, the fish become extremely agitated and their development is inhibited. Furthermore, it is highly likely that the carp louse is capable of transmitting abdominal dropsy and other diseases from one fish to another.

Clinical picture and diagnosis: Affected fish frequently show retracted fins, are very agitated and carry out scratching movements. Around the perforated areas, reddish inflammation can be observed which may develop into grayish-white discoloration. Neoplasms may sometimes form around the bite.

The carp louse (5.0–5.8 mm, about $\frac{1}{4}$ inch) can be seen quite clearly with the naked eye. It can be found anywhere on the body although it usually shows a preference for the dorsal fin. The gills may also be affected.

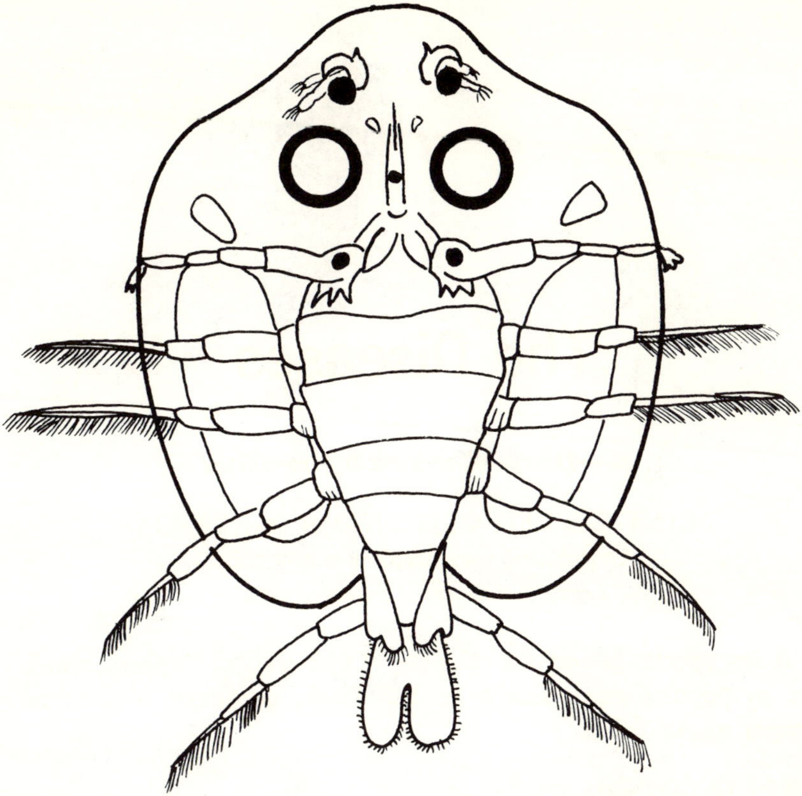

Argulus, the carp or fish louse, in ventral view.

Incidence and prognosis: Carp lice are common parasites of fishes in their natural habitat and can accidentally be transferred to the aquarium. In warm-water tanks they do not survive long. There have been occasions, however, when tropical varieties which also thrive in warm water have entered our aquaria with fish imports. Small fish can die of the toxin produced by these parasites. The disease responds well to treatment.
Therapy: Lindane; preparations containing Trichlorphon.*

GILL COPEPODS *(Ergasilus)*

Etiology: The larvae (nauplii) of *Ergasilus* (there are several

* Also commonly spelled Trichlorfon.

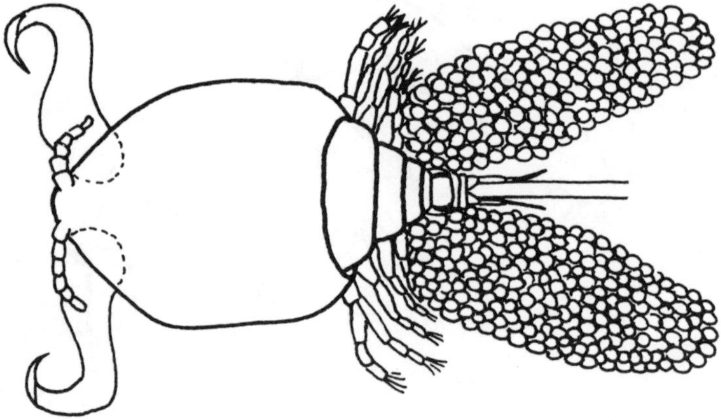

A female *Ergasilus* with large egg sacs.

Close up of the anterior part of the carapace ("head") of *Argulus*. Notice the large suckers and the median stylet of the mouthparts. Photo by Helmert.

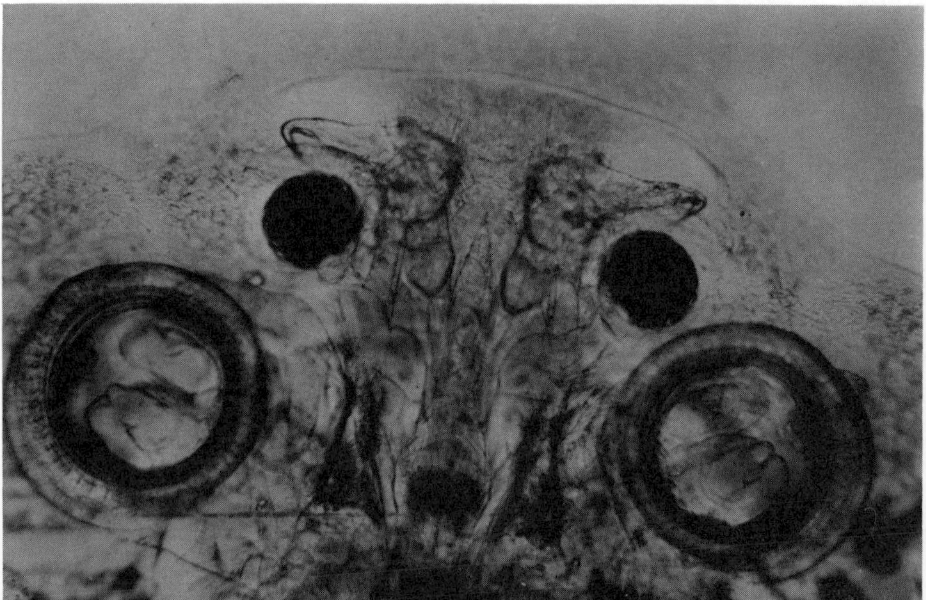

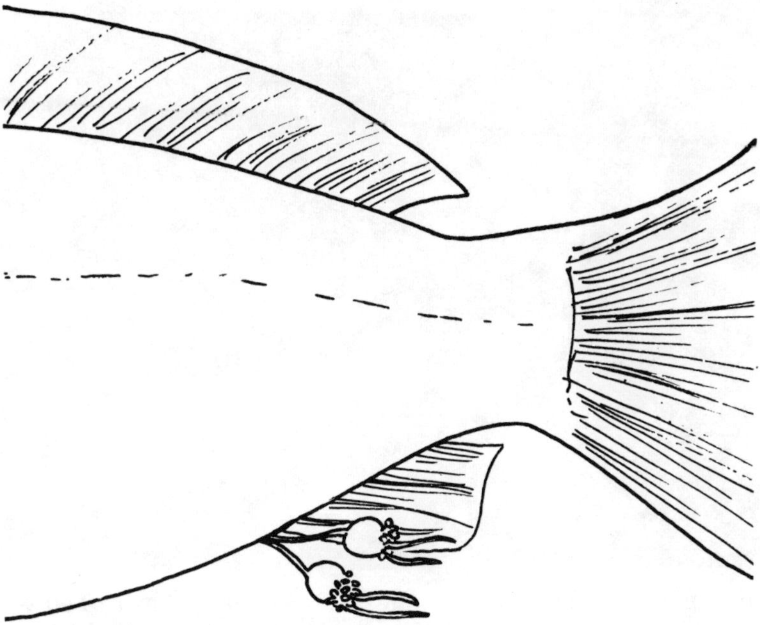

Copepods can often be identified by the shape and size of the conspicuous egg sacs, but the actual body of the parasite is often embedded in the muscles.

species) cannot be distinguished from the larvae of *Cyclops*. The nauplii of *Ergasilus*, however, attach themselves to the gills of fishes and, depending on the species, grow there to a length of up to 0.5–2.0 mm (1/50–1/12 inch). The adult crustacean does not leave the host again. With the second pair of antennae, which are transformed into hooks, the parasites cling to the gills, frequently constricting the blood vessels of the gill filaments in the process. *Clinical picture and diagnosis:* Externally the fish usually appear quite normal. If they are severely affected, however, there will be marked emaciation. The gills frequently look pale since only little blood can pass through the constricted vessels. With the aid of a magnifying glass, the crustaceans are easy to detect. Apart from infesting the gills, the parasites may occasionally be found on the skin as well. A deep blue spot on the anterior part of the body is characteristic of most *Ergasilus* species.

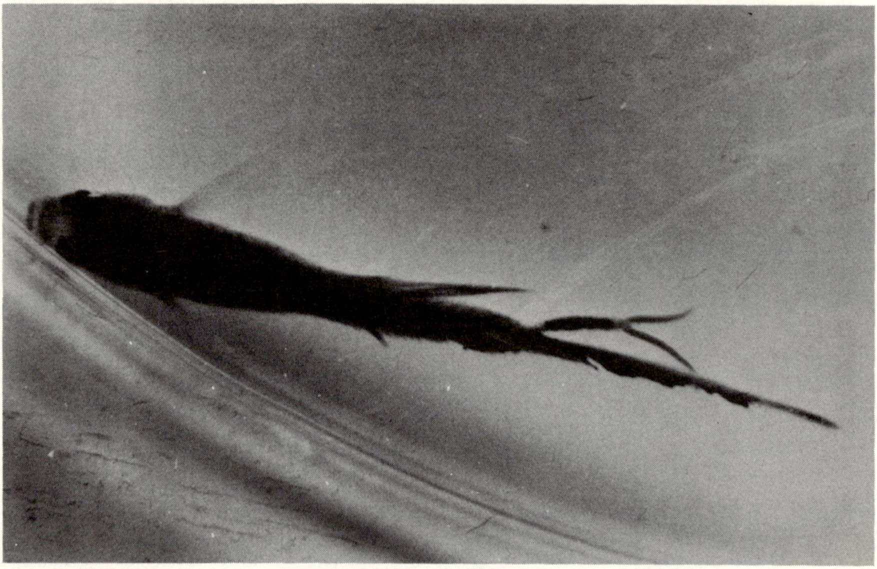

A single parasite on a large fish may do little harm, but many *Lernaea* on a small tropical fish spells almost certain death. Photo by W.A. Tomey.

Close up of the egg sacs and posterior end of two *Lernaea*. Photo by W.A. Tomey.

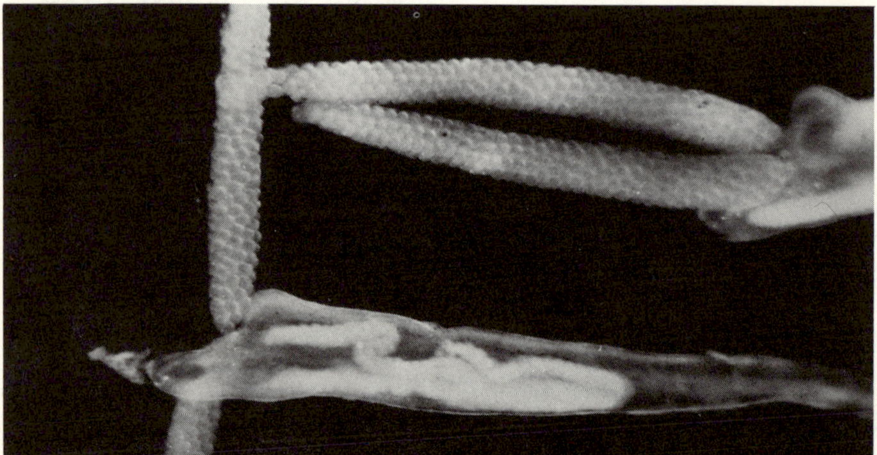

Incidence and prognosis: Ergasilus affects the larger fishes in fresh and salt water aquaria. The gills of smaller fishes do not offer support for the attachment of the crustaceans. The prognosis is good.
Therapy: Lindane; preparations containing Trichlorphon.

Lernaea AND RELATED FORMS

Species of the genus *Lernaea* and related forms vary greatly in size. The crustaceans penetrate into the skin, leaving only the large egg sacs hanging outside the body of the host. Infestation with this parasite is easily diagnosed. Recommended treatment: Lindane and preparations containing Trichlorphon.

It is easy to understand why the embedded head of *Lernaea* is often called an anchor. Photo by W.A. Tomey.

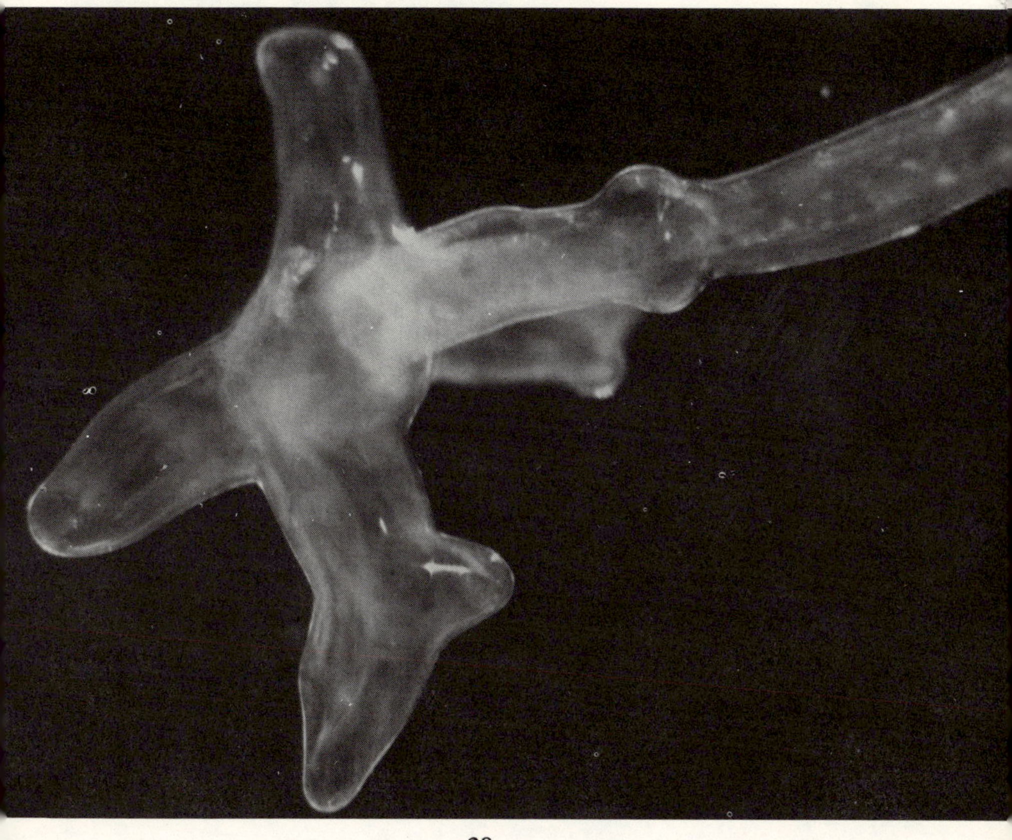

Leeches (Hirudinea)

Fish leeches, relatives of the well-known medicinal leech, can cause damage in game and food fishes. In the aquarium they are of no consequence. Most native species do not live in warm water, and their large size, 1–5 cm ($\frac{3}{8}$–2 inches), ensures that they are quickly discovered. The latter also applies to tropical species that have entered the aquarium with imported fishes. They are simply removed by hand. If necessary, immersion in a mild salt solution brings about their speedy detachment.

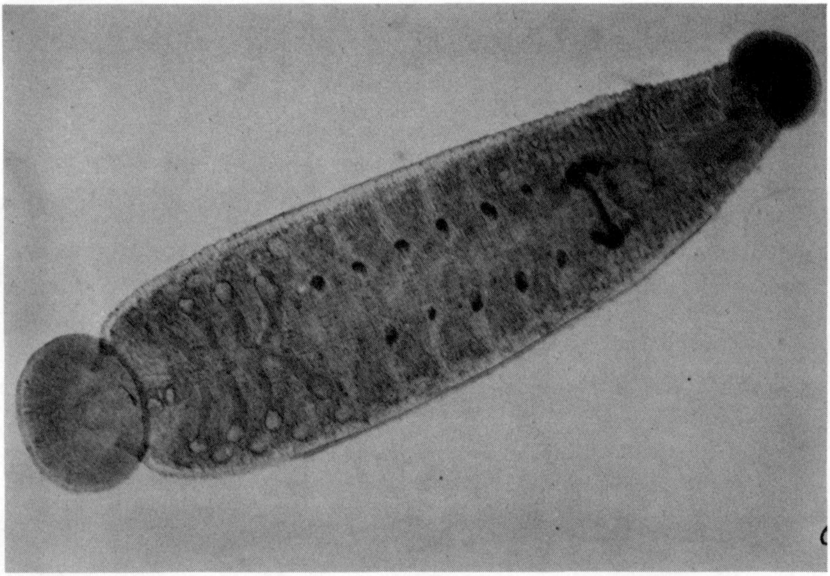

Detail view of a small leech showing the small anterior and large posterior suckers. The many sexual structures, both male and female, are also clearly visible. Photo by Knaack.

Intestinal worms (Acanthocephala).

Etiology: These parasites of the intestine are common in outdoor fishes. With their spiny proboscis they anchor themselves to the intestinal wall. The eggs leave the intestine with the feces of the host. When the larva has hatched it parasitizes small crustaceans and the larvae of insects. Any fish eating such organisms becomes infected. In some species of Acanthocephala, the first fish is needed

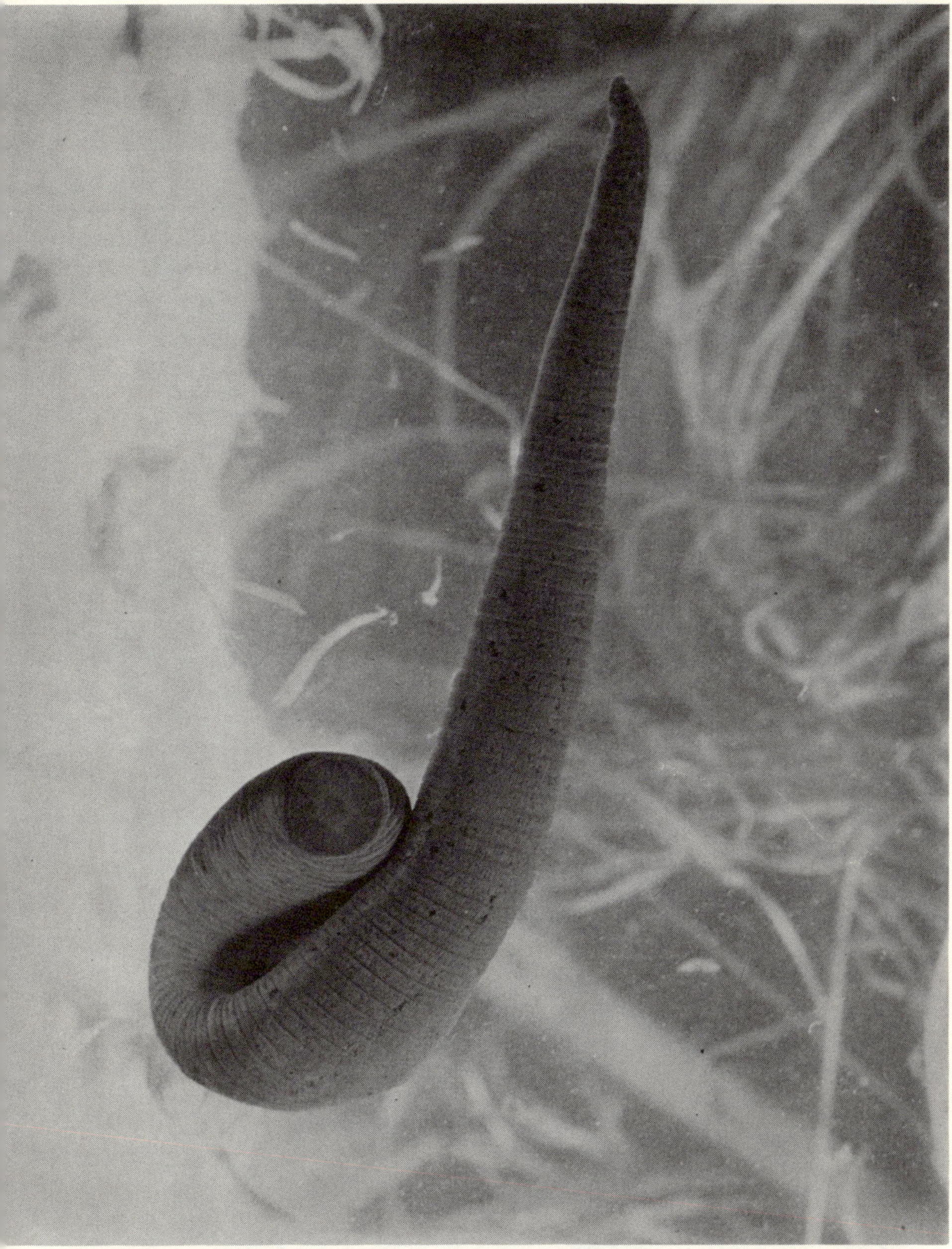

Leeches swim slowly but well, using a coiling and uncoiling motion of their elongated body. Some can actually catch small fish. Photo by G. Marcuse.

merely for the development of a second larval stage, and the adult form can only develop when this fish has been eaten by a bigger fish. Acanthocephala harm their hosts by depleting them of nutriments and, particularly, by frequently changing their location, causing injury to the intestine with the proboscis.

Clinical picture and diagnosis: The larger fishes are able to tolerate individual worms without adverse effects. Smaller fishes, or fishes that are severely infested, become emaciated and may eventually die. Adult worms are easily detected in the intestine. After the mucus has been rinsed off, their characteristic proboscis becomes discernible with the aid of a powerful magnifying glass. The larval stages of *Acanthocephalus* usually lie inside the abdominal cavity. They too can be seen to have the characteristic proboscis.

Incidence and prognosis: Acanthocephala rarely occur in aquarium fishes although wild catches may occasionally be affected.

Therapy and prophylaxis: So far a cure is unknown. There is a

The proboscis or scolex of *Acanthocephalus* is armed with many slender, curved spines. Photo by Dr. E. Elkan.

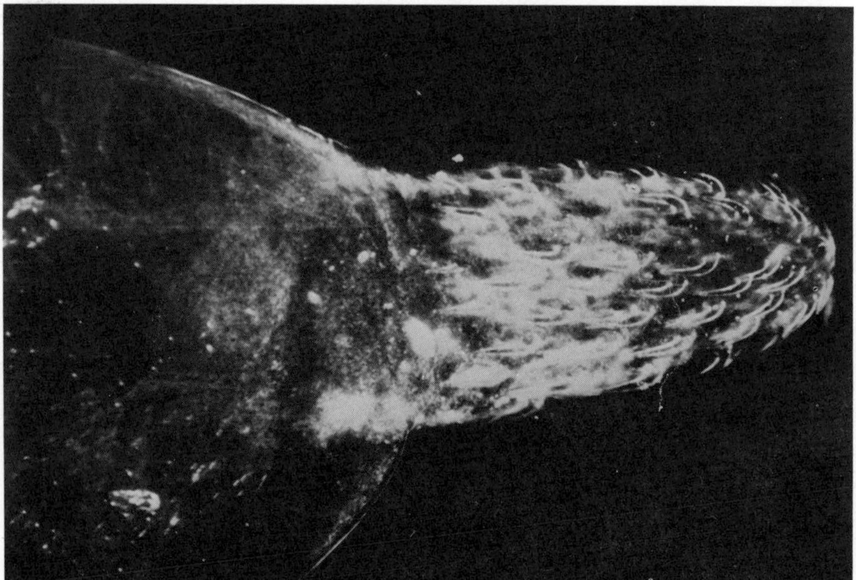

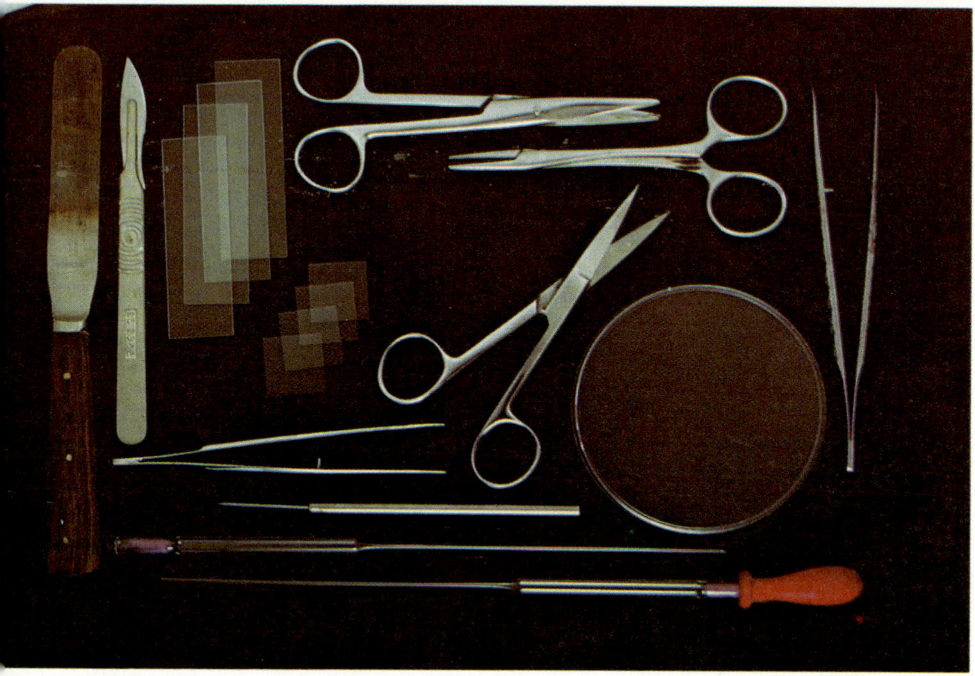

Some of the equipment used in the autopsy of a fish. Many of the items can be substituted for with common household tools.

The mature red blood cells of fishes have a well developed nucleus, unlike those of birds and mammals.

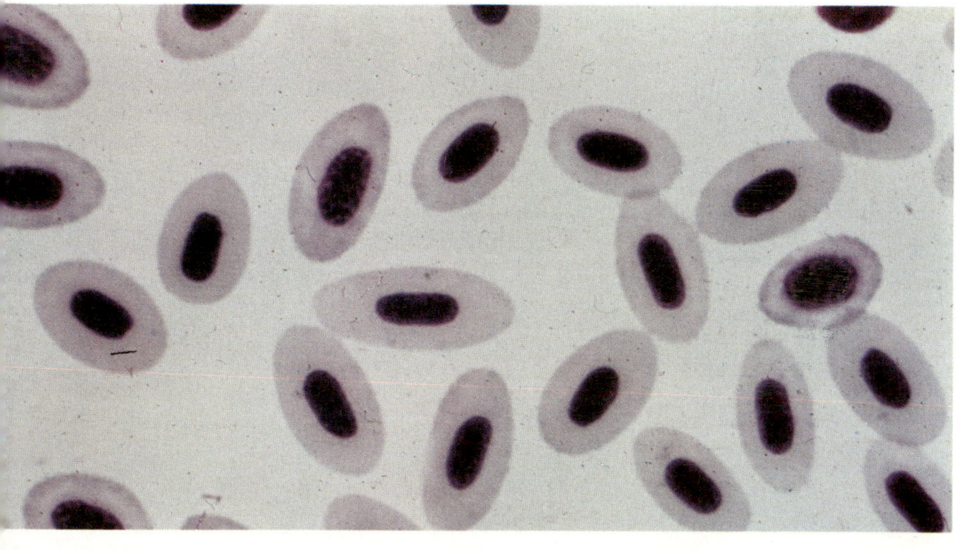

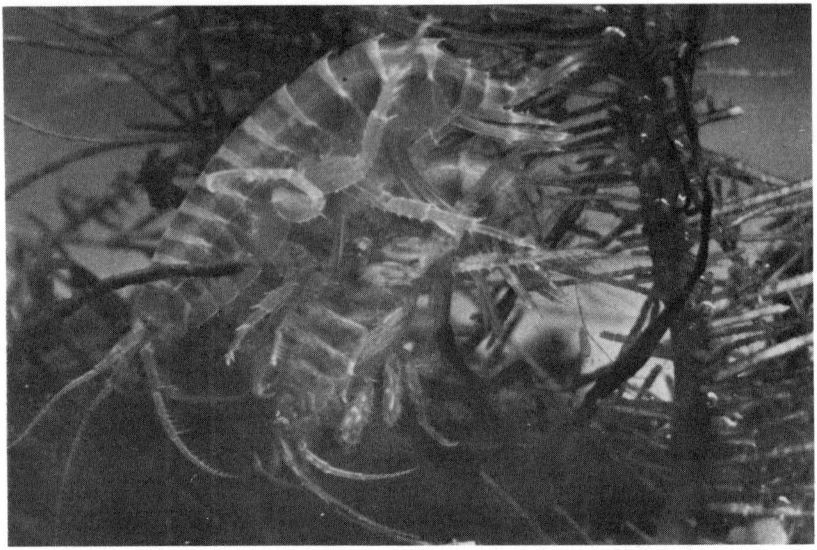

Amphipods are useful live food, but beware of those with small, scattered red spots, the larvae of acanthocephalans.

danger of larger fishes becoming infected when fed on *Gammarus* (fresh water amphipods). This excellent food should, therefore, only be obtained from waters that do not contain any fishes. *Gammarus* with small red spots (larval acanthocephala) should be discarded.

Threadworms or roundworms (Nematodes)

The majority of threadworms are very thin, and cross-sections of them always look round. Wild fishes are affected by a great variety of species which may be present as adult worms (almost always in the intestine) or as larvae (in many different organs). There the larvae wait until a piscivorous animal (a bird, a bigger fish, a crocodile, etc.) devours the fish, and it is inside this animal that they grow into the adult stage.

There is nothing one can do about the larvae. However, since most nematodes occurring in fishes need one or more intermediate hosts in order to develop, they are unable to spread in the aquarium once the developmental cycle has been interrupted. So far, only two genera that do not require an intermediate host have been found in our aquaria.

Capillaria

Clinical picture and diagnosis: A mild infection is usually tolerated without any reaction. When more severely infected, the animals suffer from loss of appetite and subsequent emaciation. The worms fix themselves to the intestinal wall and inflict considerable wounds through which intestinal parasites (e.g. *Spironucleus)* may easily penetrate into the abdominal cavity.

Infestation is quite apparent in the living animal. Newly deposited feces will be found to contain the characteristic eggs which look as though they had been sealed with champagne corks at either end. Subsequent autopsy reveals the worms, the females of which contain a large quantity of eggs at varying stages of development.

Incidence and prognosis: Capillaria is found mostly in cichlids and catfish. Angelfish, discus, and *Uaru* are affected quite frequently. A cure cannot always be achieved, and the young of infected parent animals should be reared artificially, if possible.

Therapy: The fish are fed on bloodworms which have been immersed in a solution of Concurat until the larvae were just beginning to die. Preparations containing Trichlorphon are effective in concentrations of 1.5 mg/l, but not all fishes tolerate these concentrations. It is advisable, therefore, to carry out a test on one animal to establish whether a cure is possible.

The barrel-shaped eggs of *Capillaria* are recognized by their "plugs" at each end. Photo by the author.

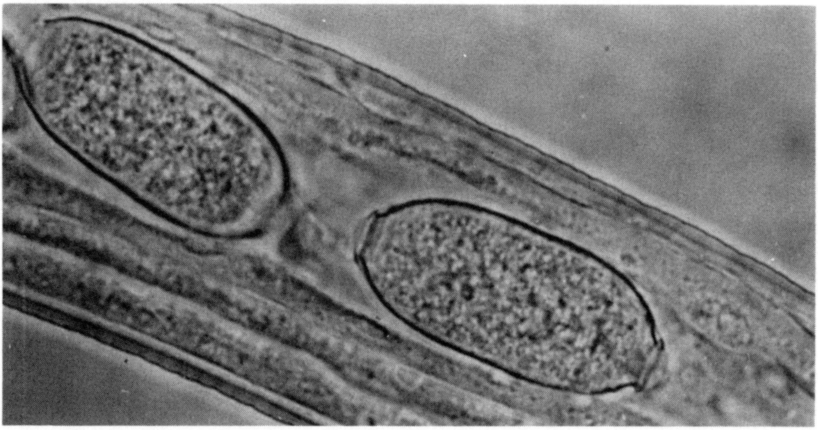

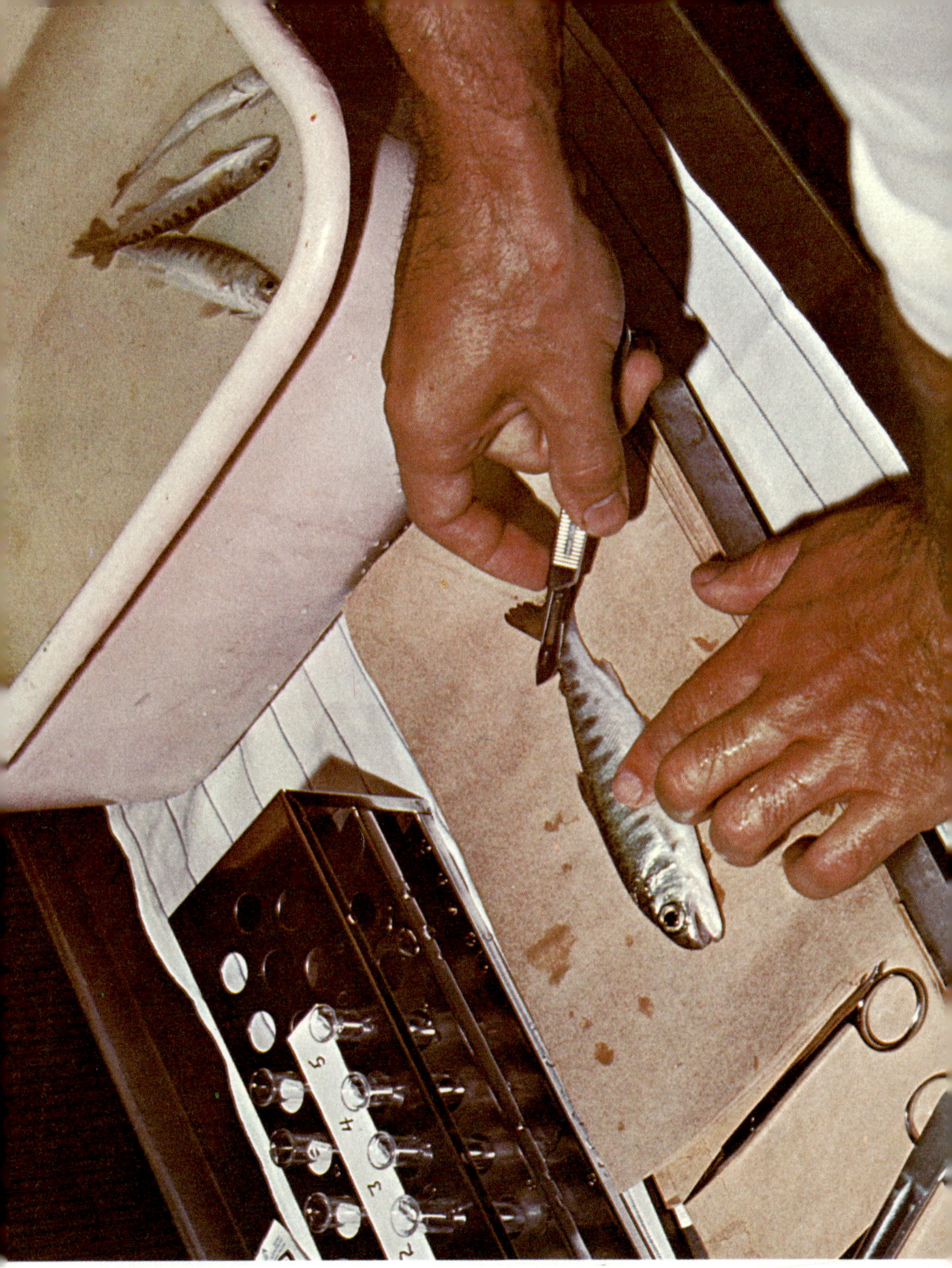

For obtaining blood from small fishes, a caudal cut is necessary. The fish is deeply anesthetized and the caudal peduncle severed. Photo by Dr. D. Anderson.

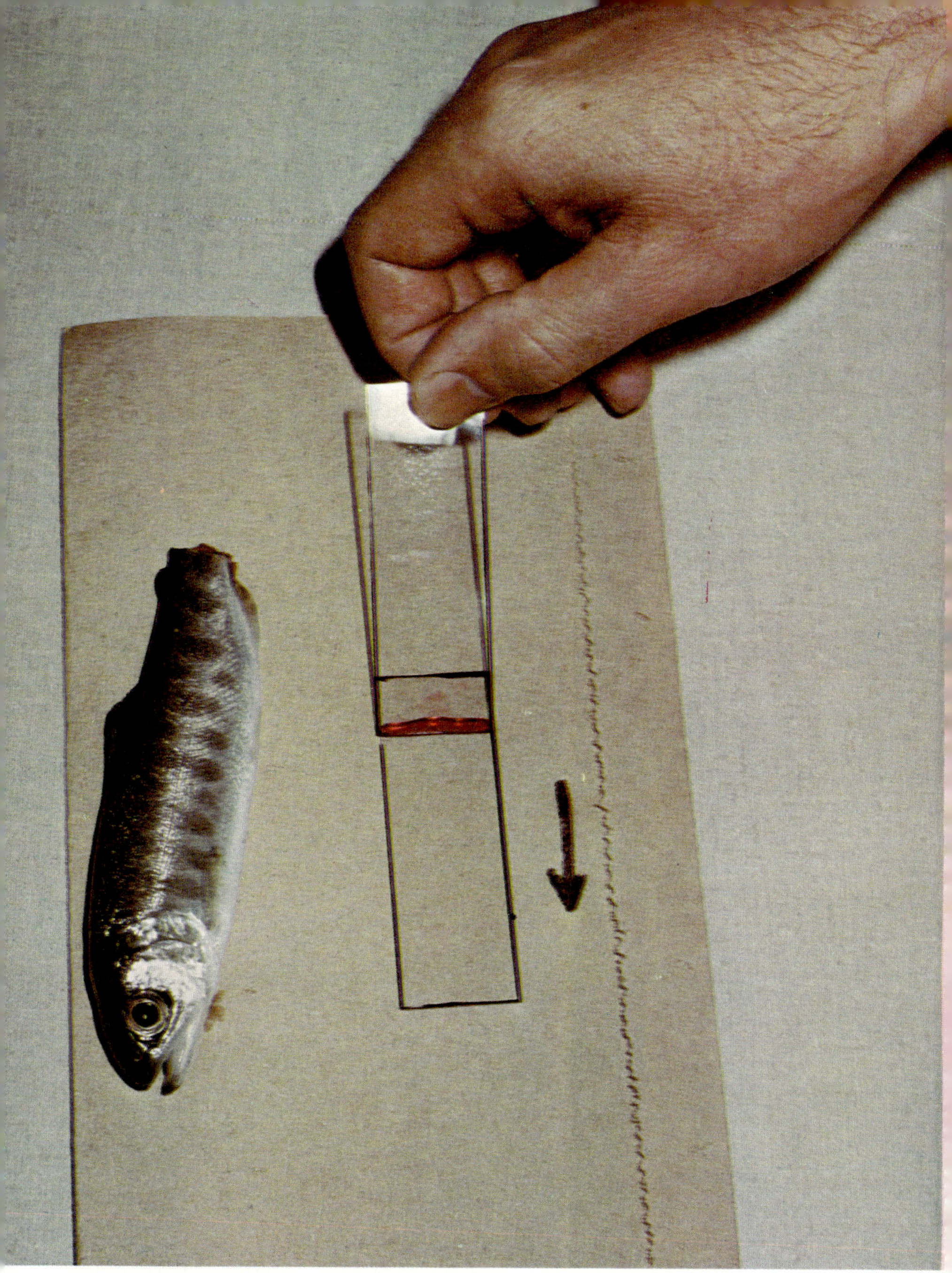

A small drop of blood is then put on a very clean slide and *pulled*, not pushed, across with a steady, rapid motion. Photo by Dr. D. Anderson.

Camallanus

Clinical picture and diagnosis: This worm lives inside the posterior end of the fish rectum. In some fish species, the deep red worms can be seen protruding from the anus by several millimeters when the fish is still, but as soon as the fish begins to move the worms quickly slip back inside. This behavior can be observed particularly where the female guppy is concerned. In other fish species the worms cannot be seen outside. However, since *Camallanus* is live-bearing, its very small and thin larvae can, with the aid of the microscope, be observed in newly discharged feces. Animals which are severely affected suffer from emaciation and frequently show curvature of the spine.

Incidence and prognosis: Camallanus can occur in almost all ornamental fishes though it is particularly common in live-bearers, especially guppies and mollies.

Therapy: Treatment with drugs containing Trichlorphon effectively removes the parasites.

Camallanus can often be seen protruding from the anus of a resting guppy, only to withdraw when the fish becomes active. Photo by the author.

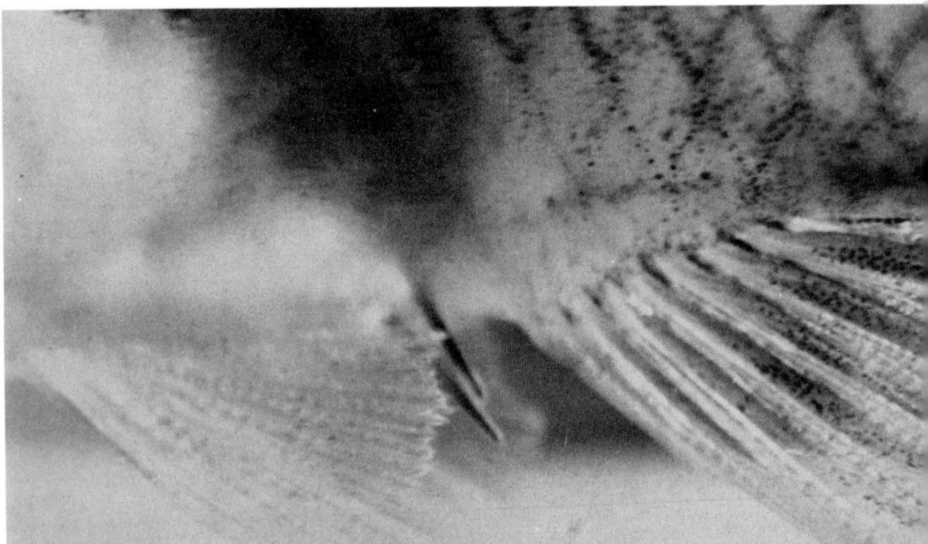

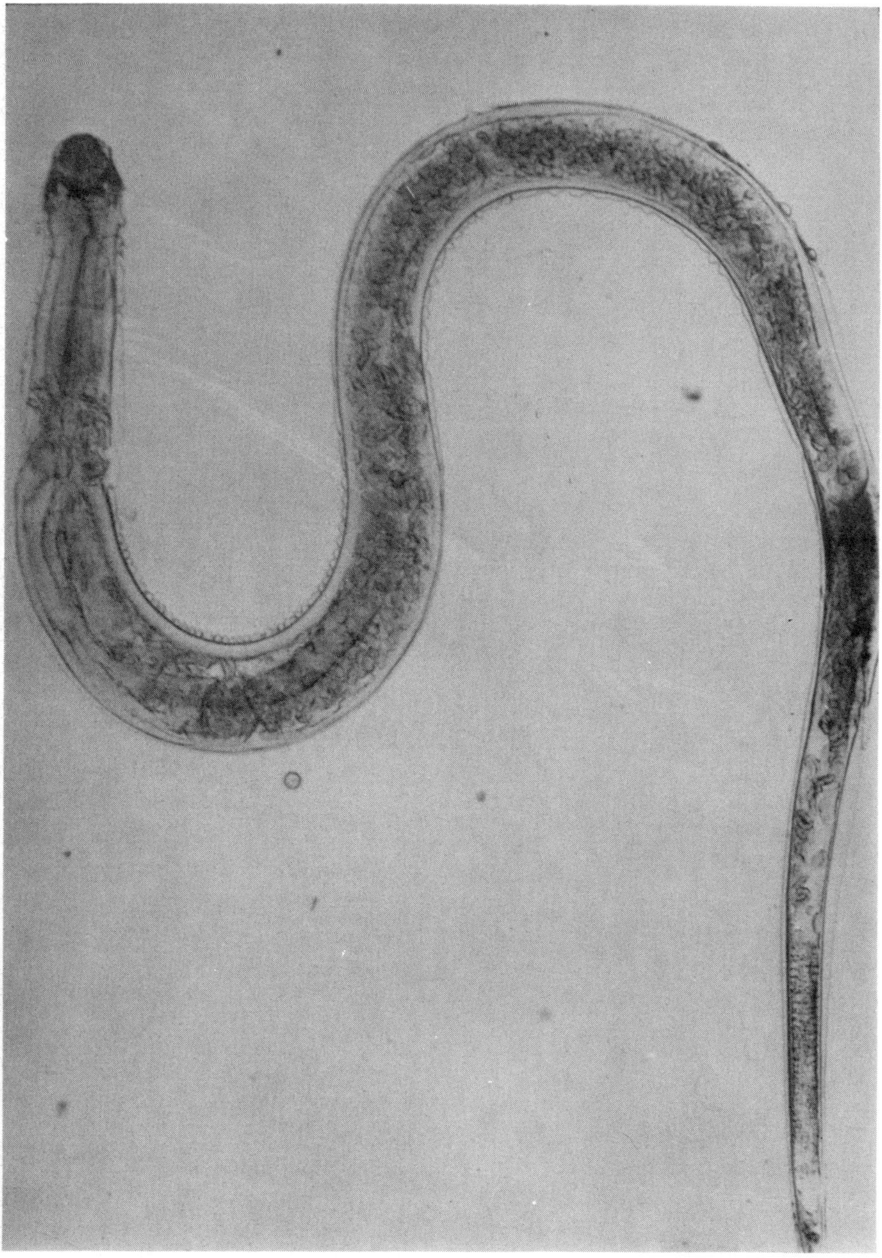

This photo of a whole *Camallanus* shows the darker head capsule and the tubular body filled with embryos. Photo by the author.

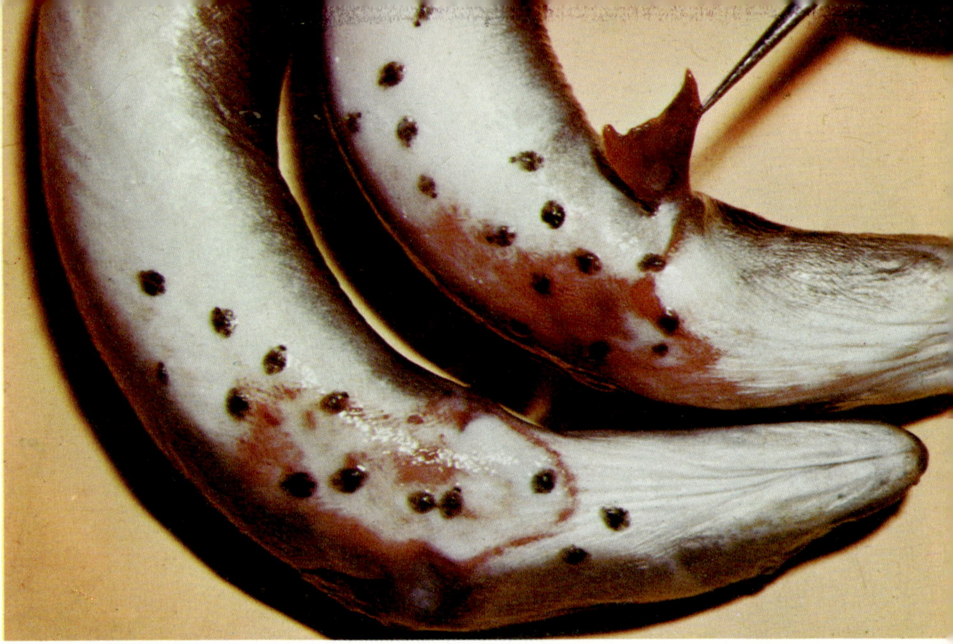

An exceptionally heavy infestation of *Argulus*. Notice the heavy rash produced by the biting and movement of the parasites. Photo by Dr. P. Ghittino.

Argulus usually attaches on the naked undersurface of the fish or on the soft tissue at the base of the fins.

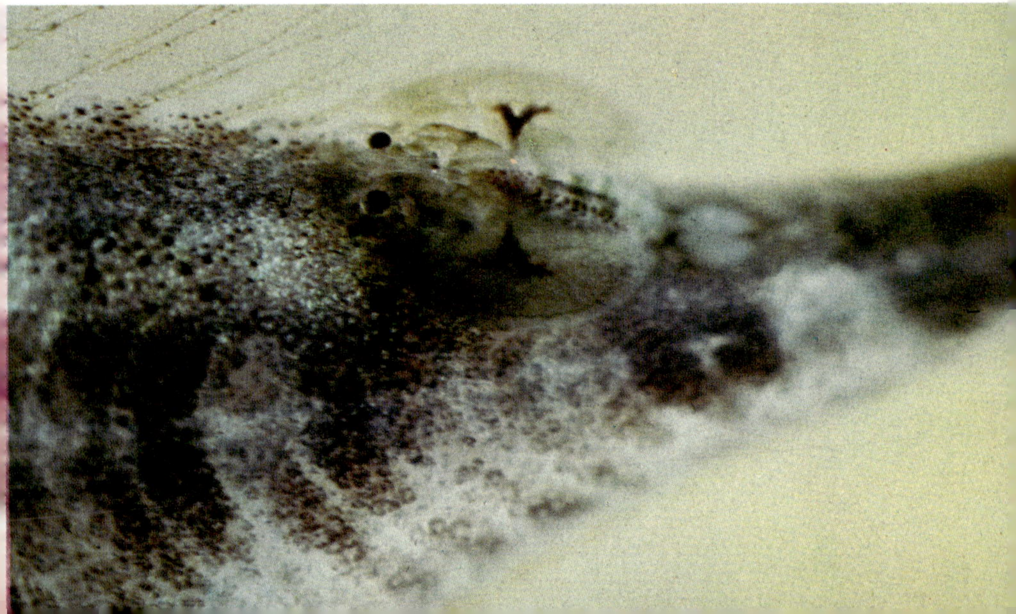

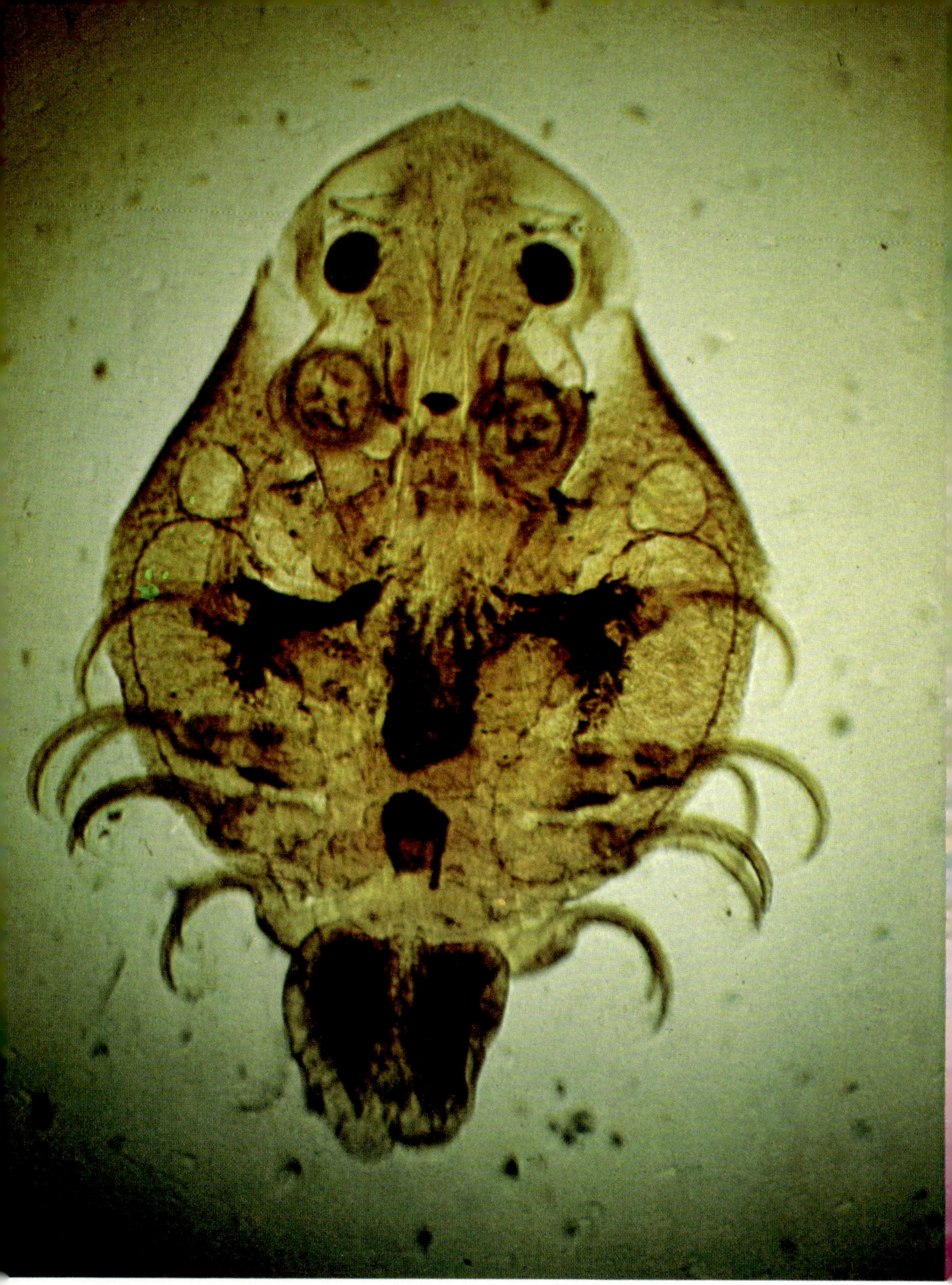

Close up of *Argulus*. Most of the parts of the body are easily visible. Photo by Dr. E. Elkan.

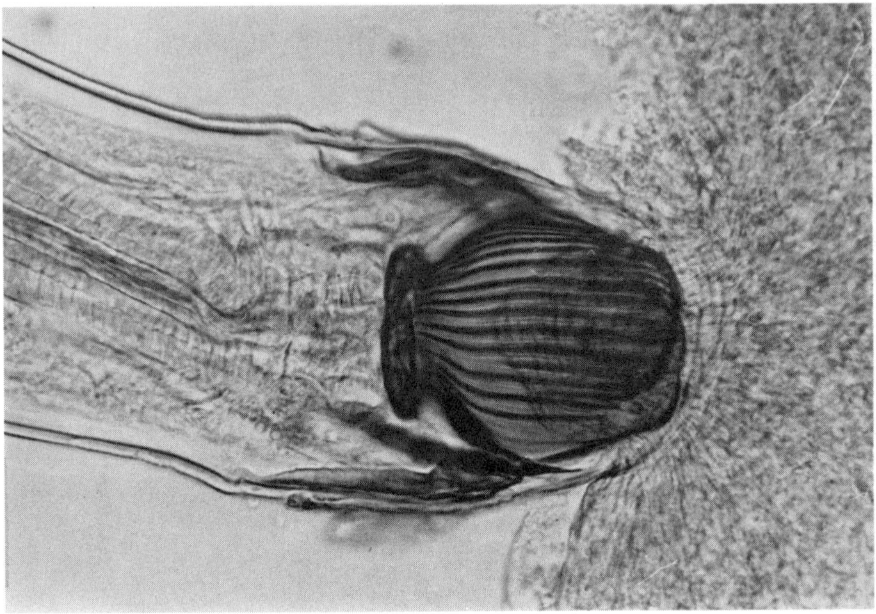

The dark "jaws" of *Camallanus* attach to the rectum and draw blood and fluids from the host. Photo by the author.

Unlike most nematodes, *Camallanus* is live-bearing, the tiny embryonic worms filling the uterus of the mother. Photo by the author.

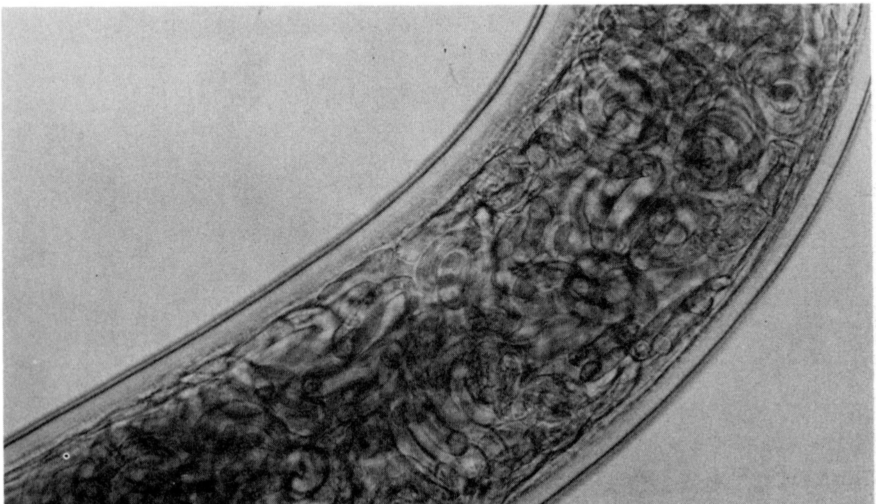

Tapeworms (Cestodes)

Etiology: Parasitism of aquarium fishes by adult tapeworms is rare and of no practical importance. *Caryophyllaeus* should be mentioned since its larvae live inside *Tubifex* and can reach our aquarium fishes with this food.

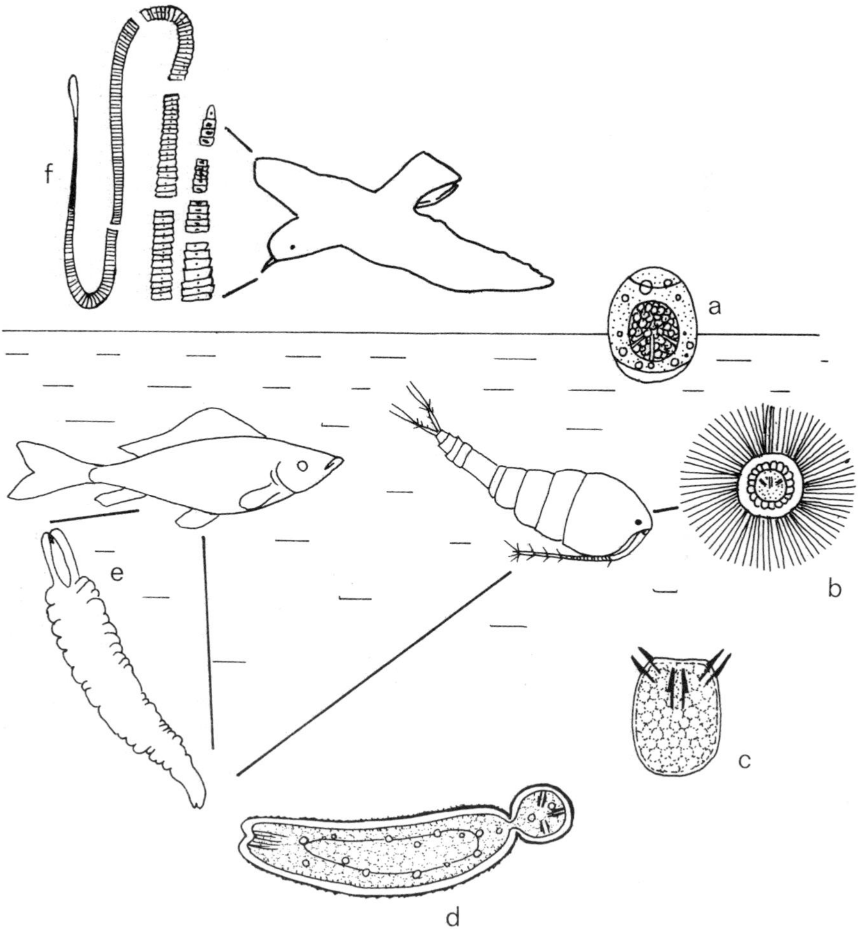

Generalized life cycle of a tapeworm: a, egg; b, coracidium ingested by copepod; c, oncosphaera; d, procercoid; e, plerocercoid eaten by fish; f, adult in bird or other final host.

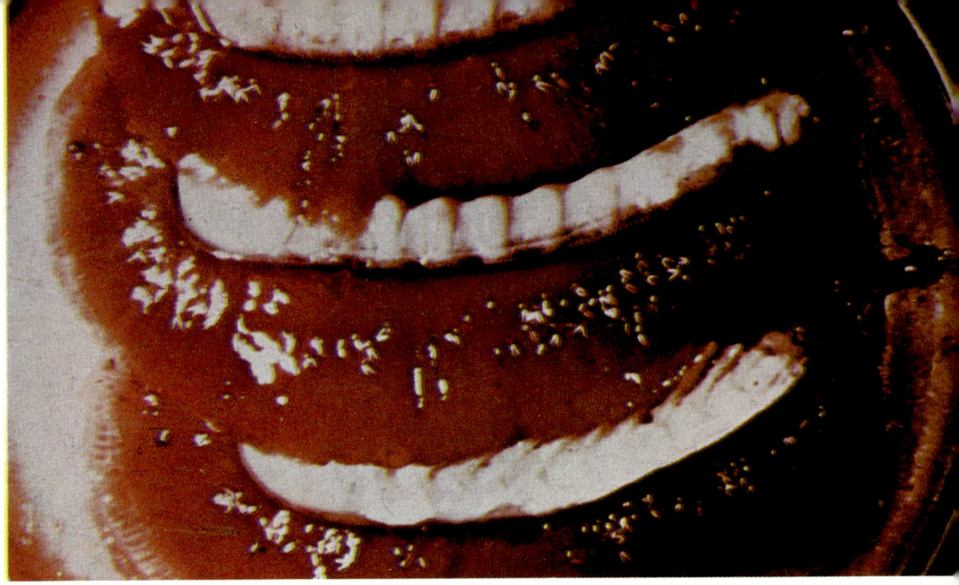

Gills heavily infested with *Ergasilus*. Notice the many small, white, inverted V-shaped egg sacs. Photo by Dr. P. de Kinkeln.

Ergasilus attached to the gills of a white crappie. Photo by Dr. F. Meyer.

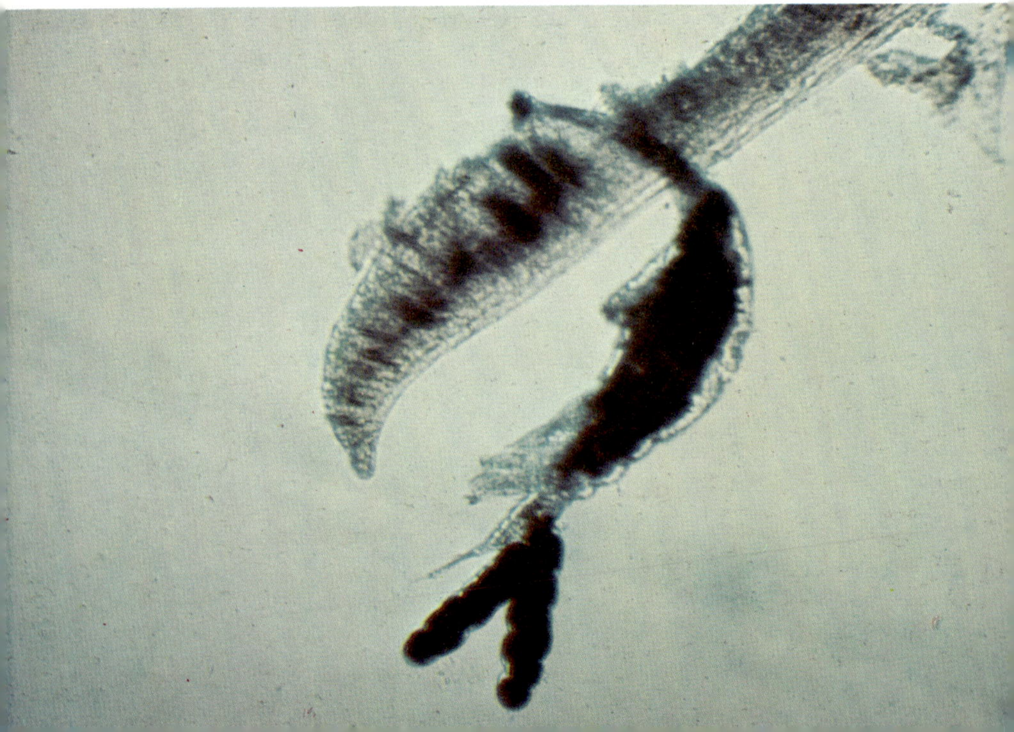

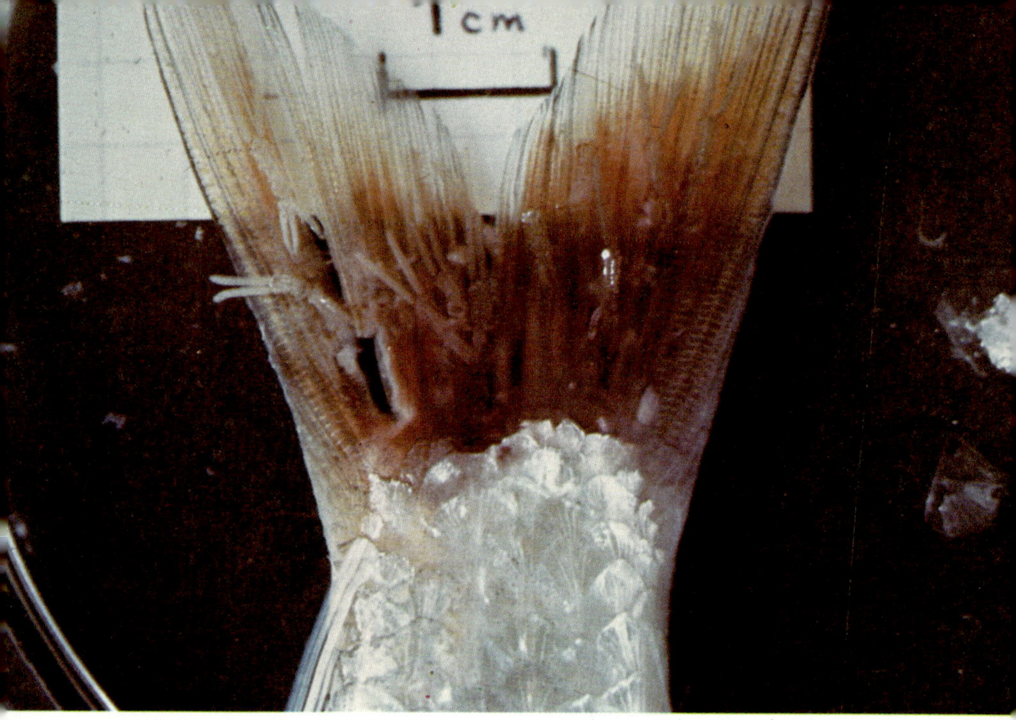

Several specimens of the copepod *Tracheliastes* attached to the caudal fin of a European roach. Photo by Dr. P. de Kinkeln.

The nauplius or early larval stage of *Lernaea*. Photo by Dr. F. Meyer.

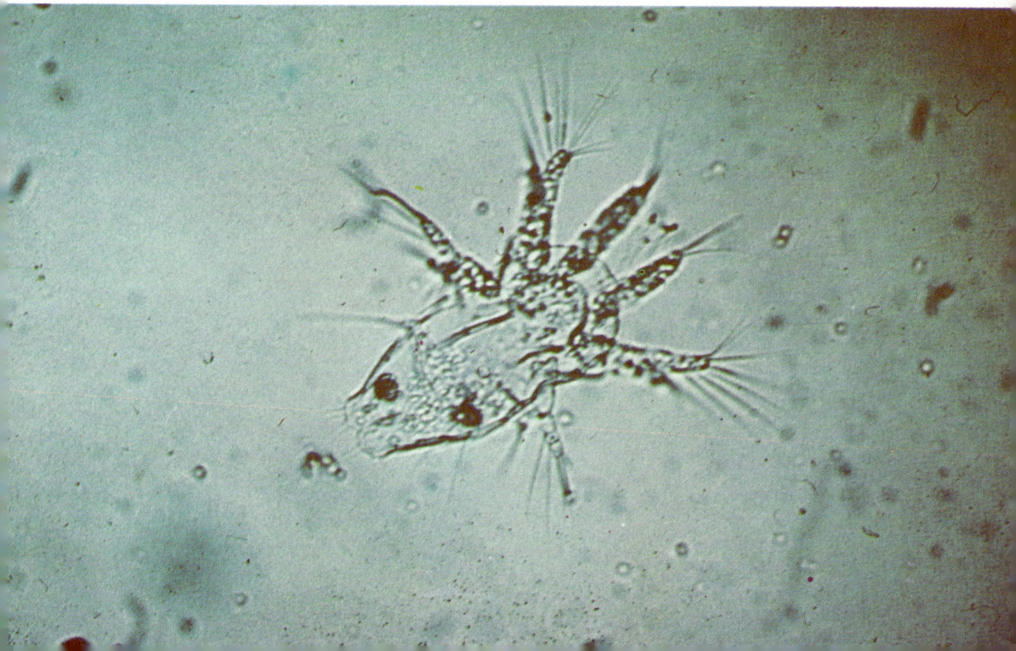

More frequently, when carrying out a closer examination, we shall observe an infestation with tapeworm larvae, which is known as *sparganosis*. The adult worms (a variety of species) live inside aquatic birds and the eggs get into the water with the feces of these birds. From the egg hatches a ciliated larva (coracidium) which is ingested by a copepod *(Cyclops, Diaptomus)*. The outer cover of the coracidium is digested and a second larva (oncosphaera) becomes free. It perforates the intestinal wall and, inside the crustacean, is transformed into a third larva (procercoid). When a fish swallows the copepod, the procercoid is liberated, migrates through the intestinal mucosa of the fish and changes into the fourth larval stage (plerocercoid or sparganum). Finally, if the fish is eaten by a bird, the plerocercoid inside the intestine of the bird develops into the adult worm.

Clinical picture and diagnosis: On dissecting the intestine, *Caryophyllaeus* immediately becomes obvious as a worm with a length of 0.8–1.4 cm ($\frac{3}{8}$–$\frac{5}{8}$ inch), broadening towards the "head." Plerocercoids, in the form of whitish or darker nodules, can occur anywhere in the body. Squash preparations reveal the suckers (bothria or attachment valves) of the adult worm. The larval stages of tapeworms frequently occur in wild catches. Treatment is not known, but the fishes do not suffer any adverse effects unless infestation is very severe.

Caryophyllaeides fennica, a tapeworm from the intestine of the European bream. Photo by Dr. E. Elkan.

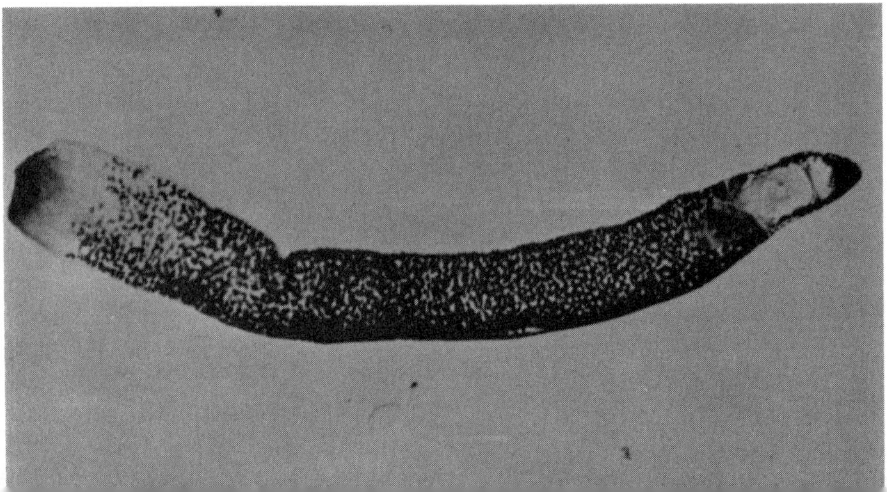

Monogenea are hermaphroditic, usually flat, parasitic worms which in their life cycle do not exhibit alternation of generations or host.

Etiology: Monogenetic worms occurring in fish are 0.05–3.0 mm (1/500–$\frac{1}{8}$ inch) long and parasitize external areas of the host's body. They fix themselves to the skin or gills with special organs of adhesion (hooks or acetabuli) and, on the basis of hook morphology, we differentiate between worms that are parasitic on the skin and worms that are parasitic on the gills. Both groups include a huge number of species which vary greatly in shape and form, and it would be far beyond the scope of this book to attempt to describe them in detail.

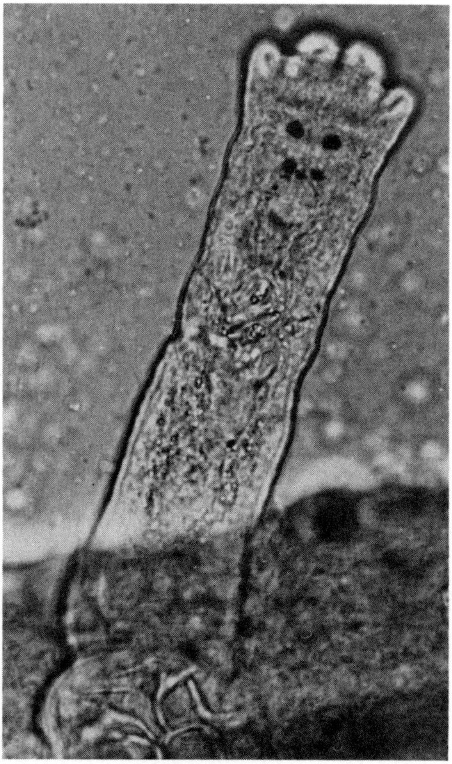

Dactylogyrus, a gill fluke or monogenea, attached to the gill of a fish. Notice the four lobes of the free end. Photo by the author.

Clinical picture and diagnosis: It is not possible for us to determine the genus, far less the species, of these worms when we come across them. But the diagnosis of skin, or gill, parasitic worms is justified

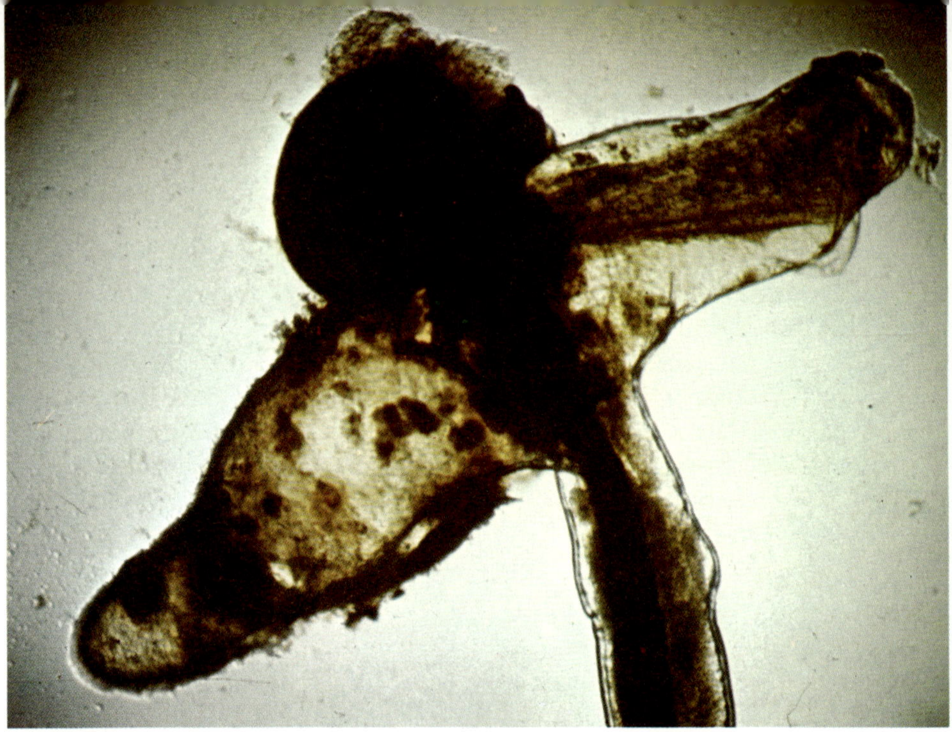

Detail of the anchor of *Lernaea*. Photo by Frickhinger.

View of an entire *Lernaea* with the egg sacs removed. Photo by Dr. F. Meyer.

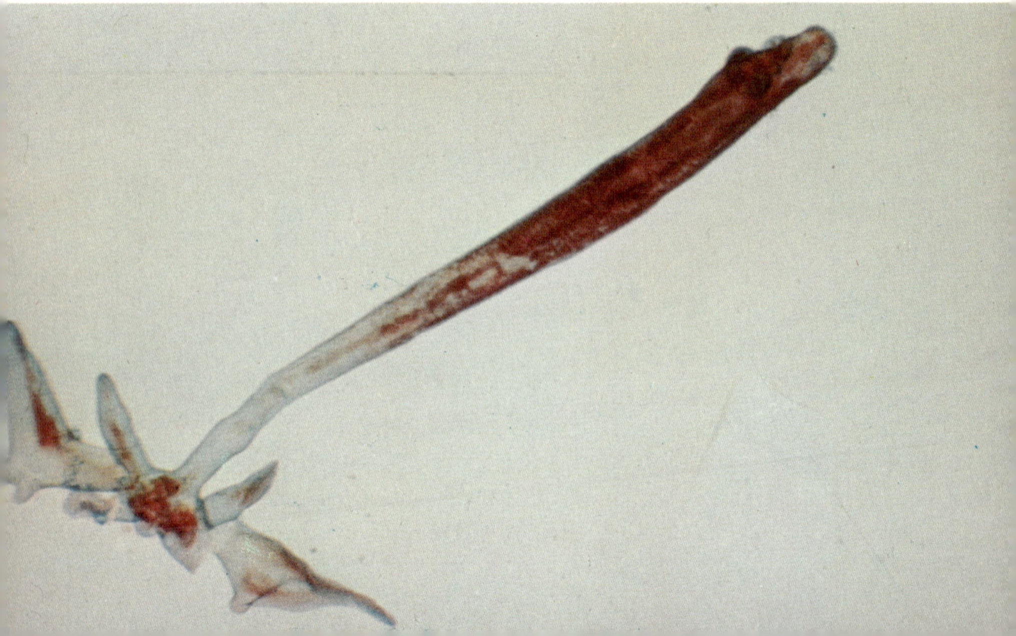

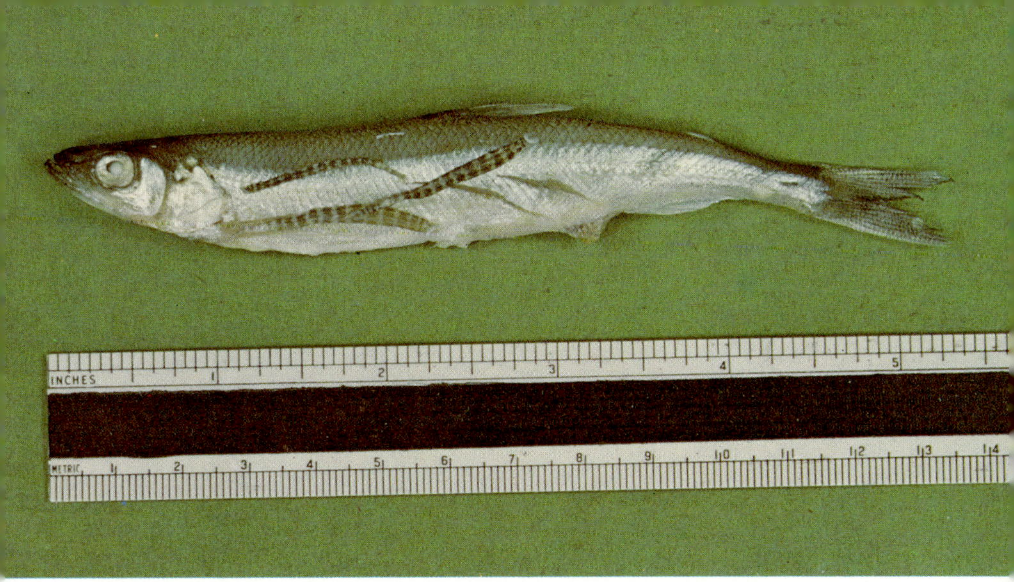

Leeches attacking a smelt. Notice the size of each parasite relative to the host. Photo by Dr. A. Dechtiarenko.

The glochidia, or larval stage, of clams can be a problem in water brought in from the wild. The little clams attach to the gills and skin of fish before dropping to the bottom and changing into adult clams. Photo by Dr. G. Hoffman.

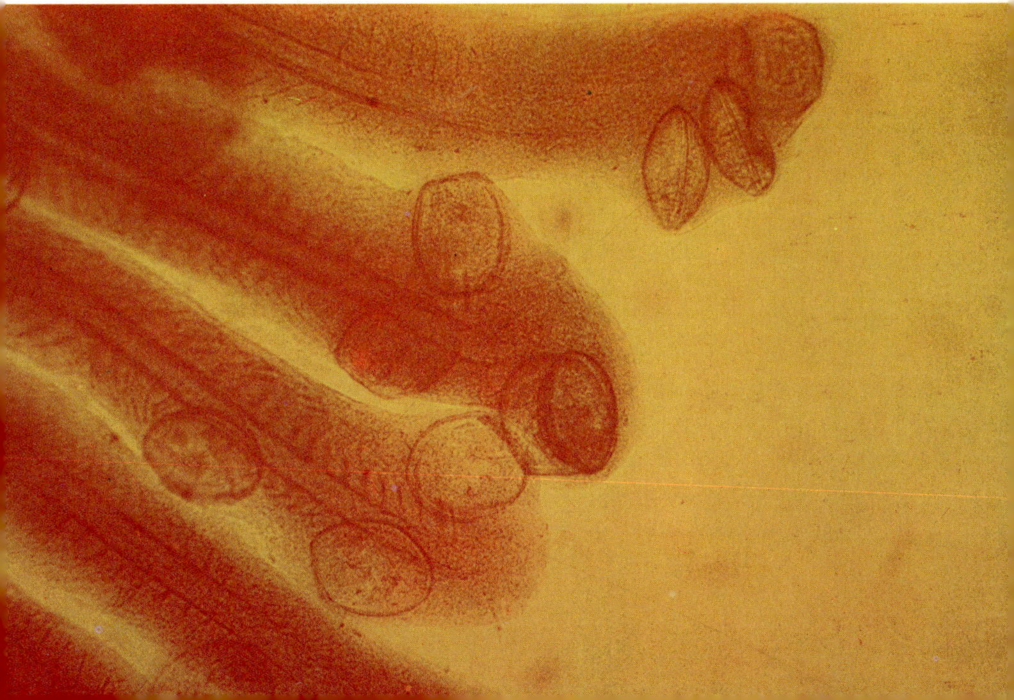

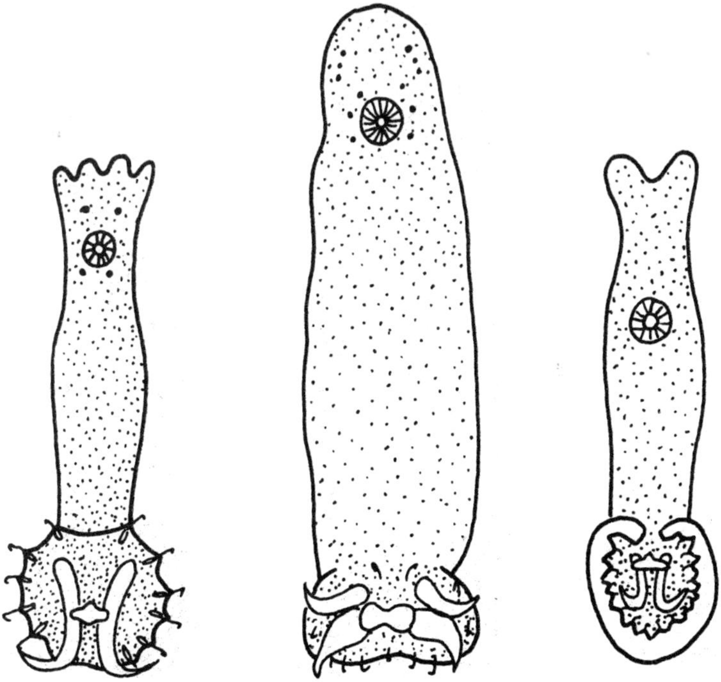

a b c

Three monogenea to show body shape and hook size. Left to right: *Dactylogyrus, Monocoelium, Gyrodactylus.*

whenever a smear taken from the fins or gills is found to contain worms which adhere with the posterior end of the body by means of hooks or acetabuli and move their free anterior end to and fro. Another important factor that has to be established before treatment can be given is whether the Monogenea concerned are egg-layers or live-bearers. The anterior end of the great majority of live-bearers has two points, but it is safer to check whether an embryo is present in the center of the worm. The embryo can be identified quite clearly by its hook apparatus. Sometimes we may also find eggs. Usually (there are exceptions) they bear long adhesive threads at one or both ends.

Affected fishes often attract our attention with their abnormally fast respiration. Faster movement of the opercula can, however, have other causes.

Incidence: Skin-parasitic worms can occur in all fishes. Gill-parasitic worms are absent in very small fishes. Frequently these parasites are specific to one host, i.e. they affect only fishes that are related. As an example, labyrinth fishes may be infected while the cichlids inhabiting the same tank remain clean, or vice versa. Particularly conspicuous is the "double animal," *Diplozoon.* Although these animals are hermaphrodites, they live permanently fused together in pairs, their bodies together resembling the letter X.

Affected with particular frequency are cichlids, puffers, certain catfishes and, among marine fishes, above all the butterflyfishes. *Diplozoon* occurs only infrequently in barbs. Gill-parasitic worms are among the most common causes of mortality in aquarium fishes.

Therapy: Short baths in salt water or formalin bring only temporary relief. Drugs based on Trichlorphon effectively combat the parasites.

Digenea

Digenea are hermaphroditic, usually flat, parasitic worms which in their life cycle exhibit alternation of generations and of hosts.

A fused pair of *Diplozoon*, the "double animal." Photo by Knaack.

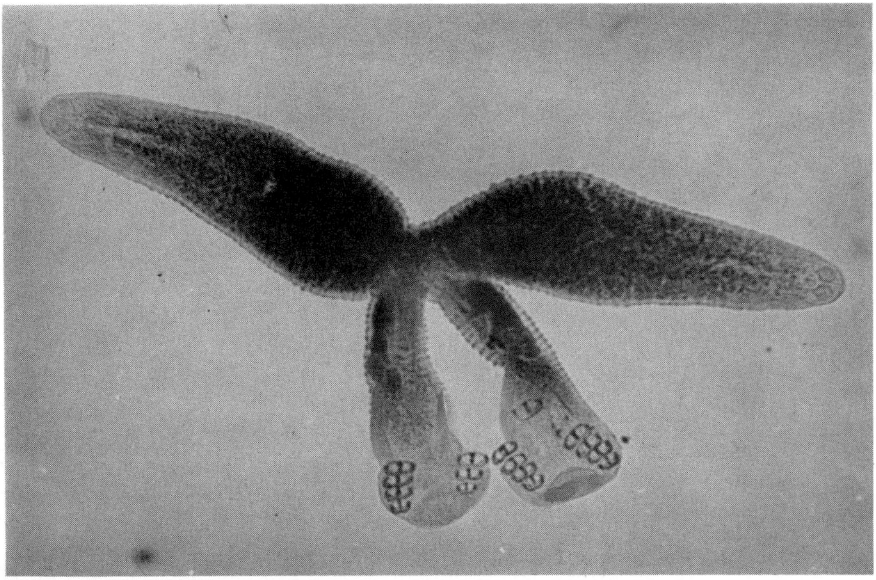

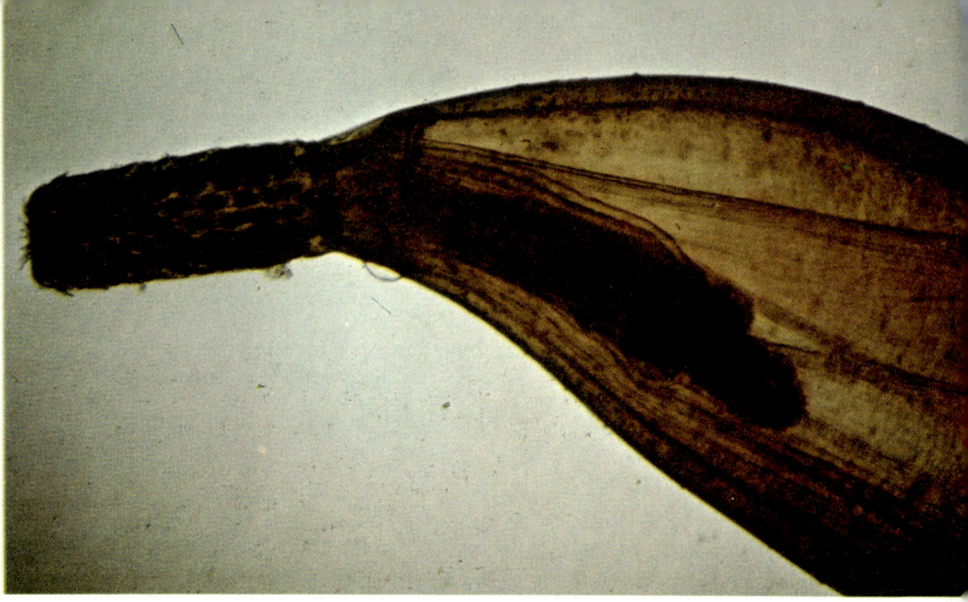

Anterior end of the acanthocephalan *Echinorhynchus*, taken from *Ctenopoma*. Photo by Frickhinger.

The number of hooks and their shape are important in distinguishing the species of acanthocephalans. This is *Leptorhynchoides thecatus*. Photo by Dr. G. Hoffman.

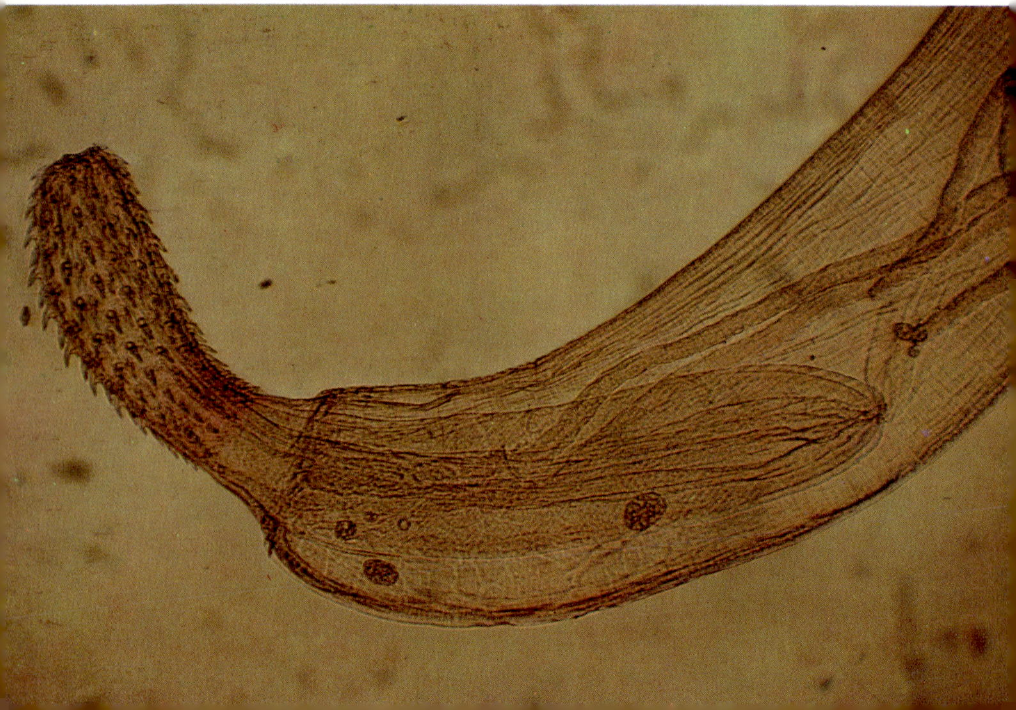

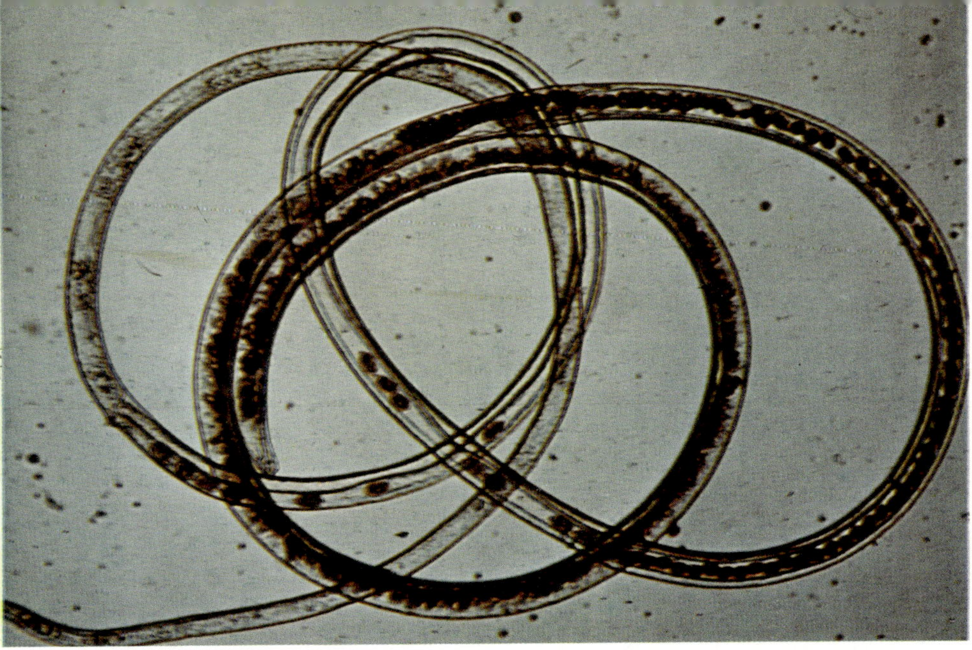

Capillaria, the thread worm. Taken from the puffer *Tetraodon palembangensis*. Photo by Frickhinger.

Larvae of the red nematode worm, *Eustrongylides*, are often found attached to the organs of fish. Photo by Dr. A. Dechtiarenko.

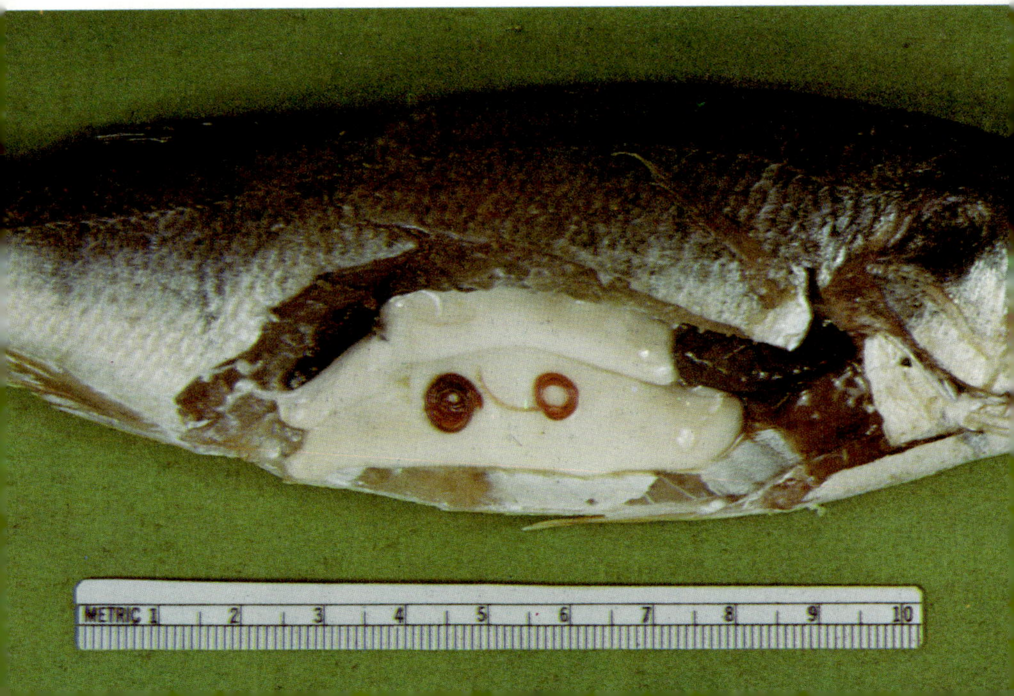

DISEASES CAUSED BY METACERCARIAE

Etiology: Digenetic trematodes have a complicated life cycle. In species which are pathogenic to fish, the adult worm generally parasitizes the digestive tract of a piscivorous bird. The eggs are expelled into the water with the feces of the host. A microscopic ciliated larva (miracidium) hatches and penetrates the body wall of a snail. In the liver of the snail the miracidium is transformed into a second larval stage (sporocyst) inside which numerous rediae (first generation) are formed. Inside each redia are now produced numerous cercariae (the larva of the adult worm). The cercariae leave the snail and penetrate the skin of a fish, losing their tail in the process. In the tissue of the fish they become encapsulated (= metacercariae). The cycle is completed when a bird ingests the fish and the metacercaria grows into the adult worm (second generation).

Clinical picture and diagnosis: Metacercariae form small black or reddish nodules under the skin, and occasionally in other organs as well, which are particularly conspicuous in the eye. Infestation with metacercariae can result in muscular atrophy and paralysis; in the eye it can lead to blindness. General disturbances of the metabolism may also occur. When we dissect an infected eye or examine teased preparation of the muscle, we often find round to oval metacercariae showing suckers and a Y-shaped intestine.

Diplostomum spathaceum, a trematode which often invades the eyes of fishes.

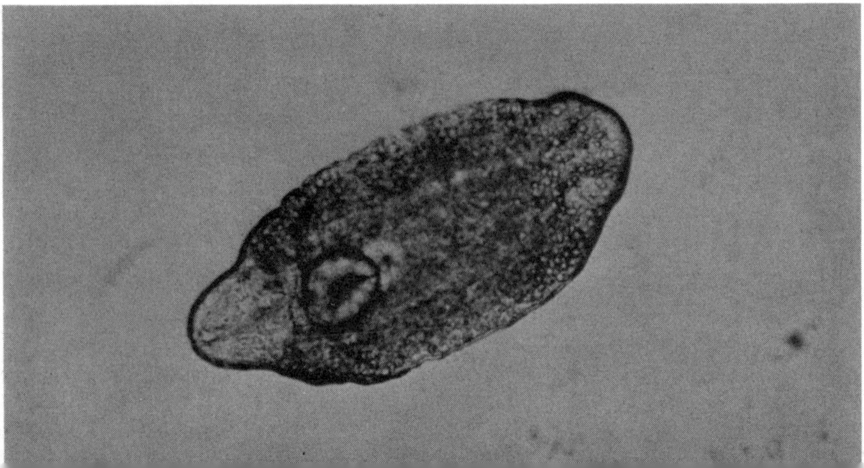

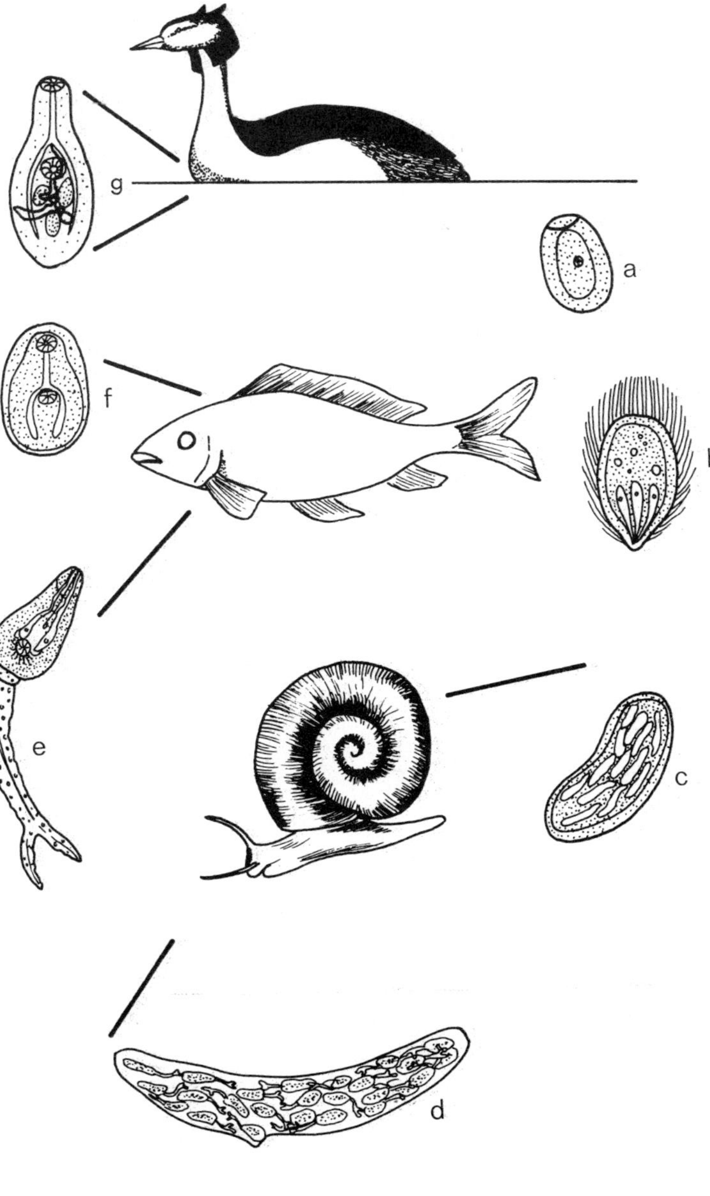

Life cycle of a digenetic trematode: a, egg; b, miracidium; c, sporocyst in snail; d, redia, also in snail; e, cercaria; f, metacercaria in fish; g, adult trematode in fish-eating bird.

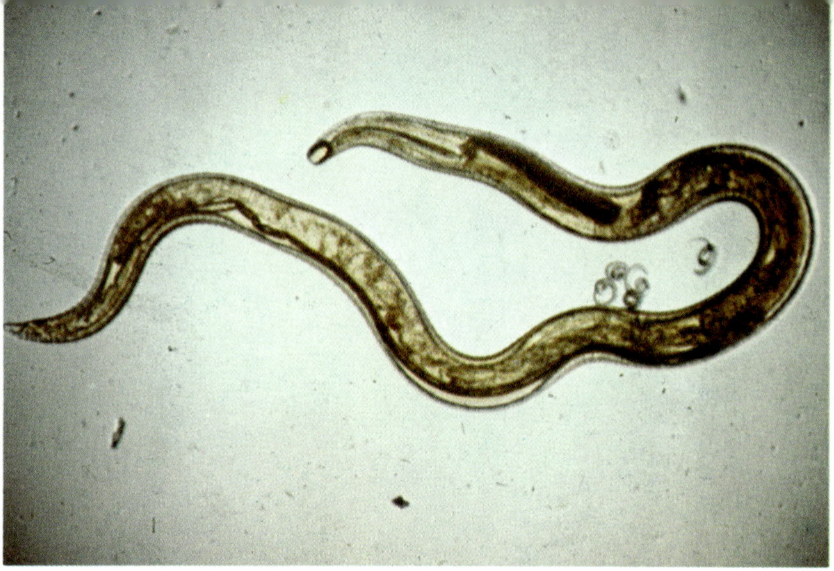

Philometra, a nematode which gives live birth to its young. Notice the five young being born. Photo by Frickhinger.

Philometra may be found in the body cavity of the fish or even in surface cavities such as mucous channels. Here it is in the cheek cavity of a sucker. Photo by Dr. G. Hoffman.

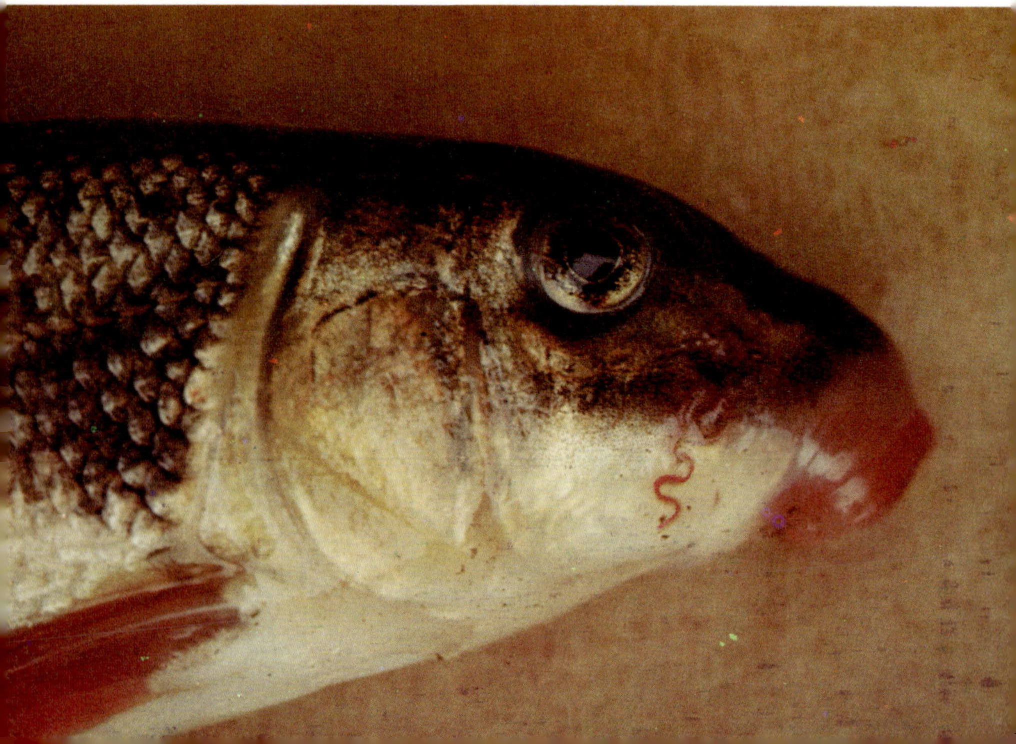

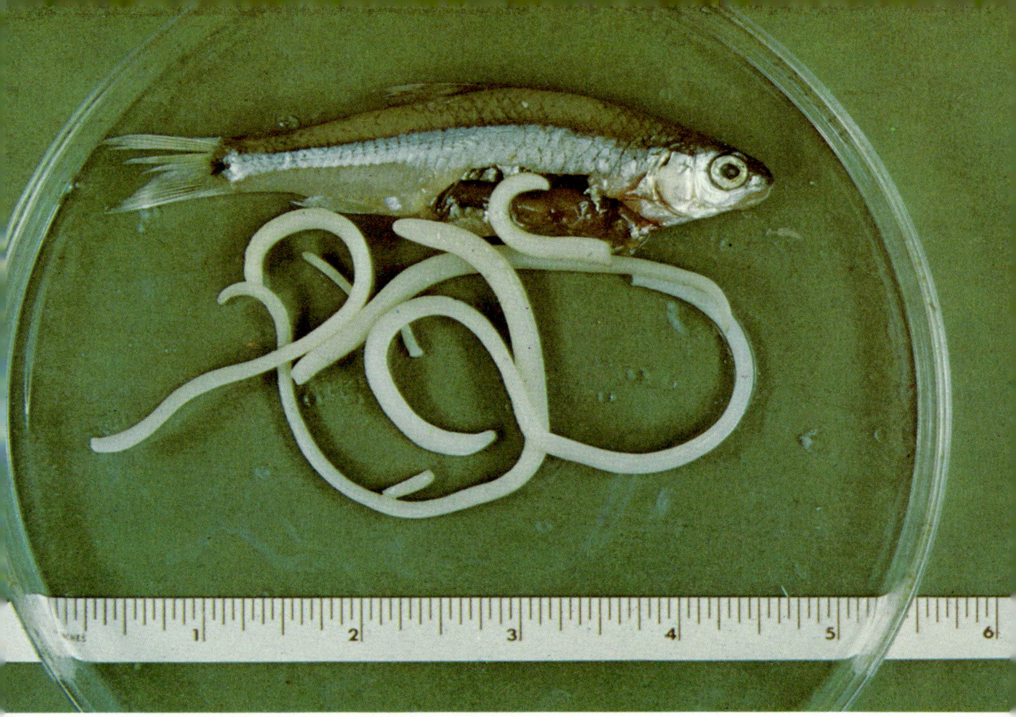

Some tapeworms, such as this *Ligula intestinalis*, can reach large sizes in even small fishes. Photo by Dr. G. Hoffman.

Although most tapeworms have conspicuous reproductive segments or proglottids, not all species have the segments as distinct as these *Eubothrium salvelini*. Photo by Dr. L. Margolis.

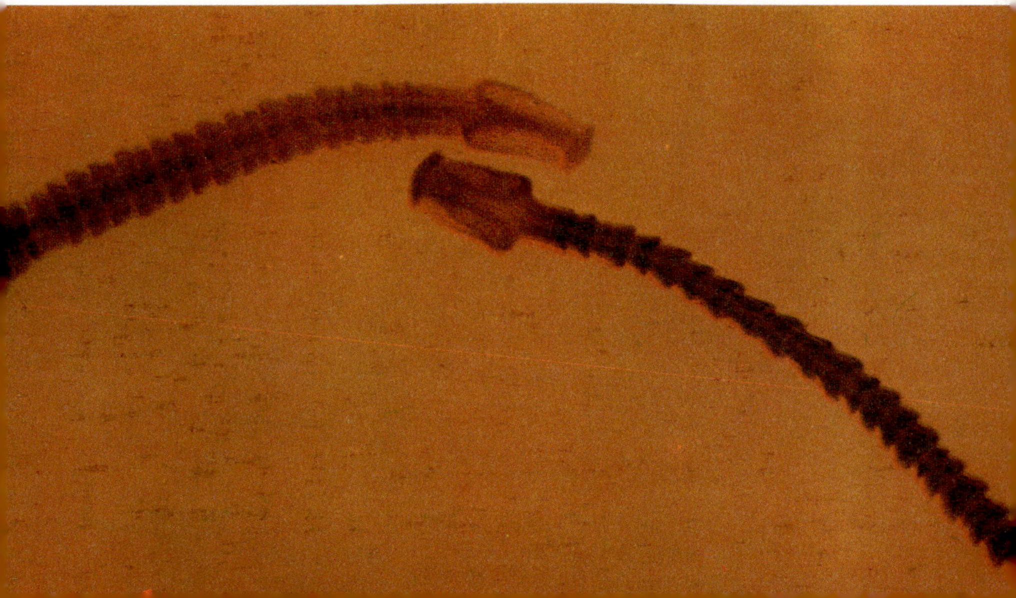

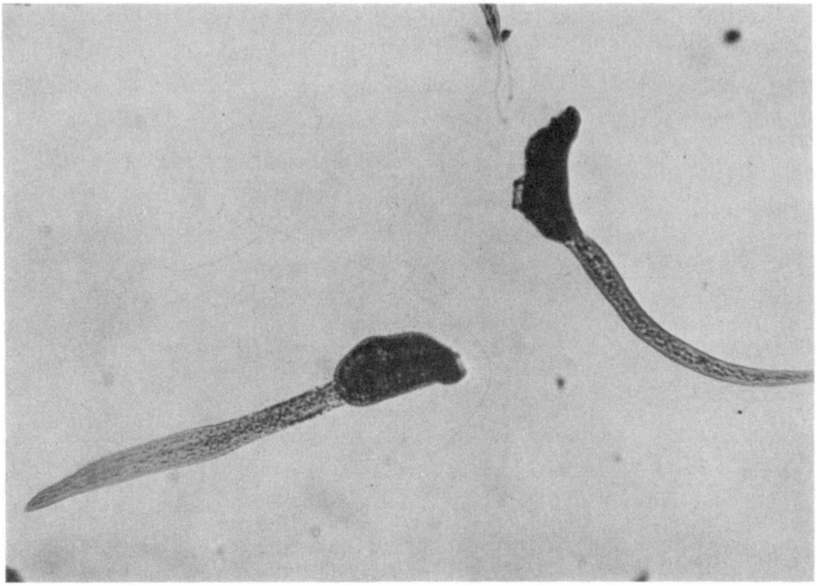

Typical cercariae have a long tail of a different consistency than the body; the tail is soon lost. Photo by Knaack.

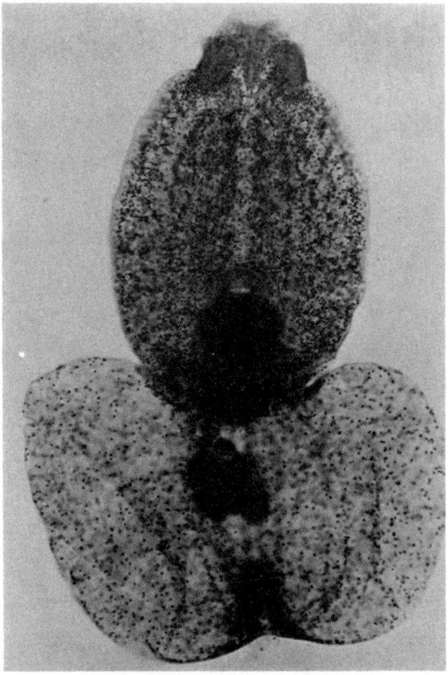

Some fluke larvae have unusual tail shapes, such as this specimen from the intestine of a discus, *Symphysodon*. Photo by the author.

Incidence and prognosis: The disease is found almost exclusively in imports. An infection of the fish can only occur via snails. Snails from outdoor waters do not belong in the aquarium, regardless of whether the waters they come from are inhabited by fish or not, since birds, other intermediate hosts, can get everywhere. Snails that have been raised in the aquarium cannot be infected. Imported fishes should be carefully examined before a purchase is made. A cure is not possible.

THE BLOOD FLUKE, *Sanguinicola*

Etiology: The adult blood fluke lives inside the blood vessels of fishes, its eggs being carried to different parts of the body by the blood. If they reach the gills, a ciliated larva (miracidium) pierces the egg and the host's tissues and escapes into the water. Its subsequent development is similar to that described under DISEASES CAUSED BY METACERCARIAE, except that the cercaria entering the fish grows into the adult worm inside the fish's blood vessels.

Tricornered egg of the blood fluke, *Sanguinicola*.

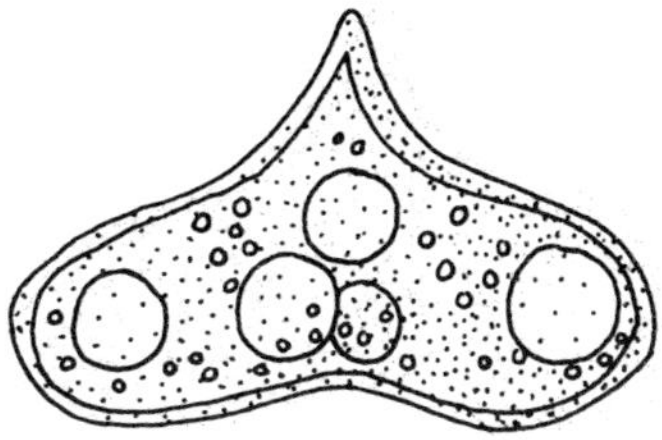

Clinical picture and diagnosis: The host is damaged mainly by the eggs, which can obstruct the capillaries. Frequently this results in the partial death of some of the host's organs, especially the gills. For diagnostic purposes, we have to make teased and squashed preparations of gills, liver and kidney. These will be found to contain characteristic hat-shaped eggs. They are fairly small, measuring about 70 microns in diameter. Occasionally, dead eggs surrounded by connective tissue may be found.
Incidence and prognosis: The disease is rare in aquarium fishes. If it has been carried into the aquarium, the remainder of the fishes can only be infected if snails are present in the tank. There is no cure for this disease.
Therapy: None. Where the disease has been diagnosed, all the snails in the aquarium have to be destroyed.

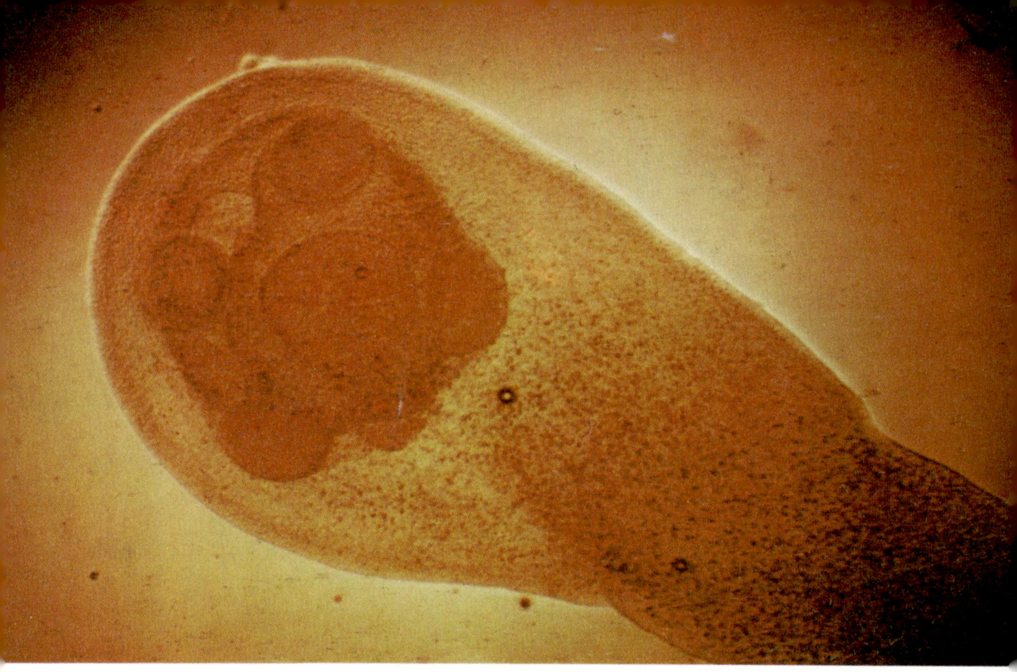

Plerocercoid of *Proteocephalus*, showing the scolex with four suckers. Photo by Dr. W. Rogers.

The white, worm-like plerocercoid of *Diphyllobothrium* passing through the liver of a salmon. Photo by Dr. R. Dexter.

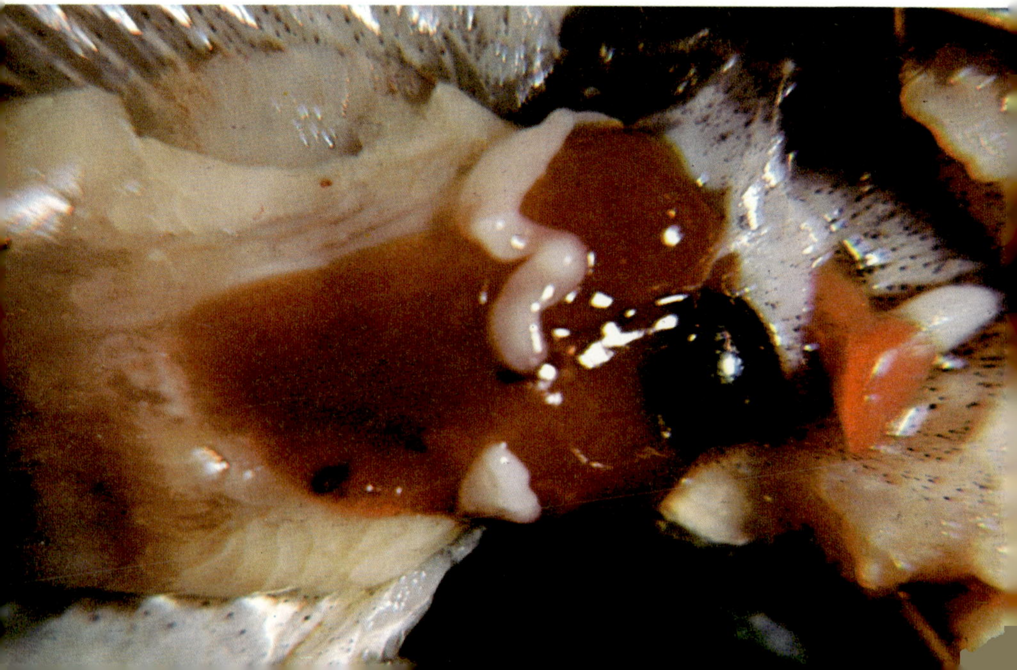

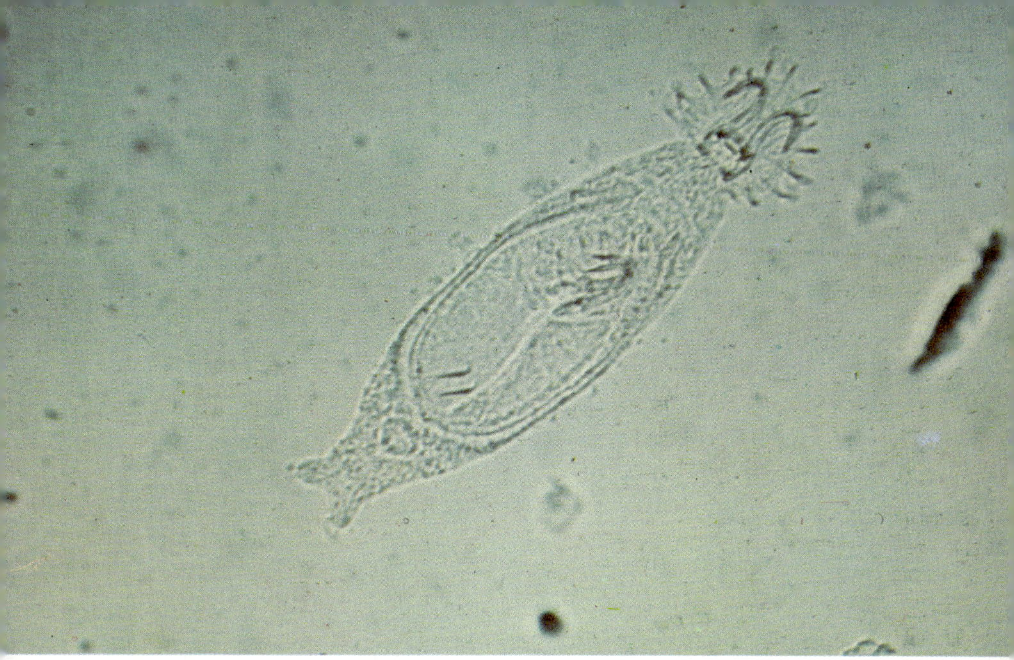

The gill fluke *Gyrodactylus*. Photo by Dr. F. Meyer.

Heavy infestation of *Dactylogyrus* on the gills of a small minnow. Photo by Dr. W. Rogers.

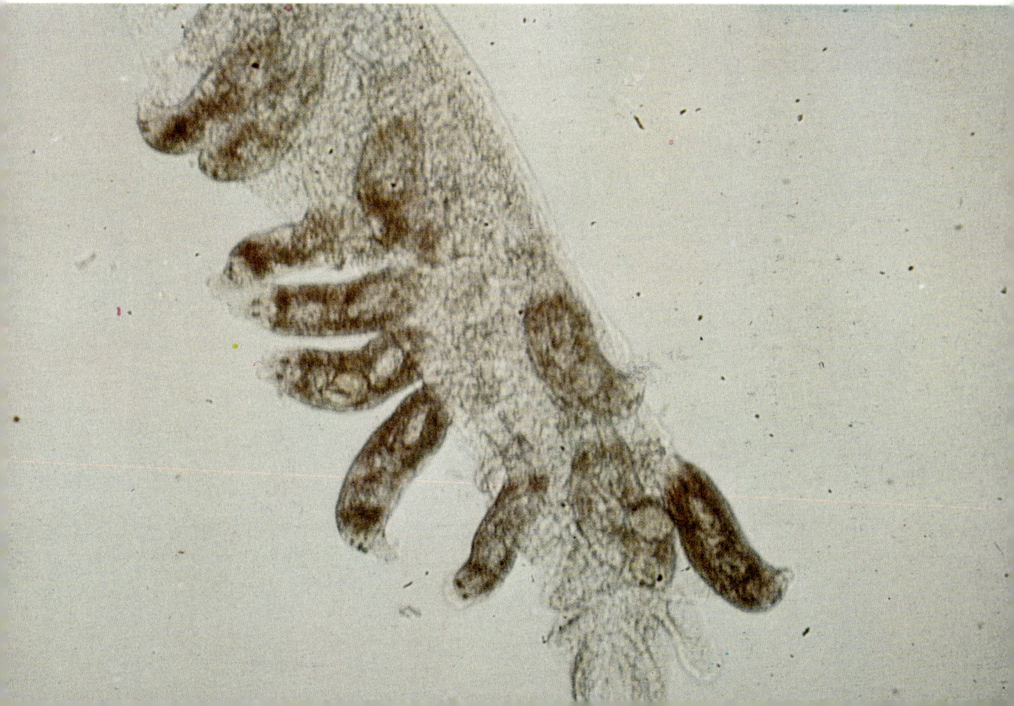

PROTOZOANS

Organisms consisting of a single cell.

Flagellates

Unicellular organisms with one or more locomotory flagella.

Costia

Etiology : Costia, the small bean-shaped causal agent of skin turbidity, is a minute flagellate with 2–4 flagella. It parasitizes the skin and occasionally the gills of fishes. In the absence of a host it quickly dies.

Clinical picture and diagnosis: Fishes suffering from costiasis show a soft, film-like skin turbidity which looks less solid than that caused by other skin parasites. However, since *Costia* frequently occurs in the company of other causal agents of skin turbidity, thicker deposits may also be observed. Severely affected areas may be inflamed and hence of a reddish appearance. Infected fishes often show swaying movements and are seen to scrape themselves against solid objects. Like most causal agents of skin turbidity, *Costia* is a "debility parasite" in that it affects only fishes that have already been weakened by other causes. Healthy, robust fishes are rarely affected. Young fishes constitute the highest risk group. The diagnosis is based on the microscopic examination of skin and gill smears. For this, greater magnifications (at least 300 times) are necessary.

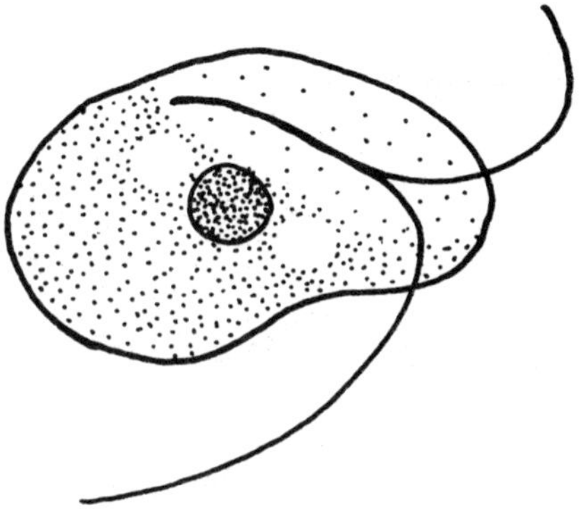

Costia, showing two flagella.

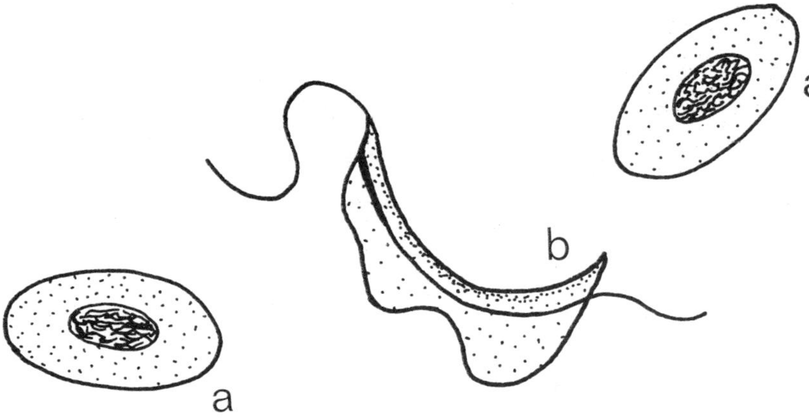

The flagellate *Cryptobia*: a, red blood cells; b, free flagellate in blood stream.

Without the aid of specific staining techniques, the layman will usually detect nothing more than small, quickly moving organisms. Since all other causal agents of skin turbidity become quite visible at medium magnifications, the presence of marked skin turbidity and the absence of other causal agents make it very likely that *Costia* is responsible.

Incidence and prognosis: In the aquarium, *Costia* is a frequent cause of the unsuccessful rearing of fry. Particularly susceptible to the disease are young killiefishes. With the exception of veil-bearing forms, adult fishes, provided they are strong and healthy, are not at risk.

Therapy: If *Costia* is the sole cause of the signs, raising of the temperature to 30–32° C (86–90° F) usually proves successful, provided the fish can tolerate it. The only chemical method of treatment that can be recommended is long duration baths in malachite green.

Cryptobia

Etiology: The "sleeping sickness" of fishes is caused by *Cryptobia*, a flagellate that lives in the blood. The disease is transmitted from one fish to another by fish leeches.

Clinical picture and diagnosis: Affected fish grow very listless. In

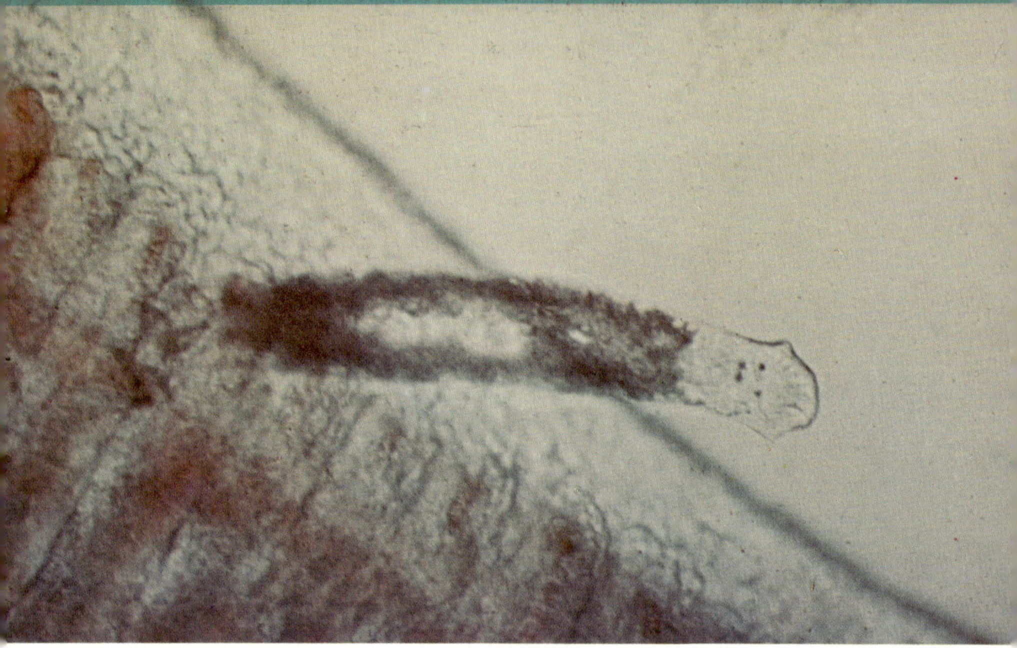

The fluke *Cleidodiscus*. Notice the rounded head end with large eye-spots. Photo by Dr. F. Meyer.

The trematode (or fluke) *Crepidostomum* is a digenea. Notice the absence of hooks and eye-spots. Photo by Dr. G. Hoffman.

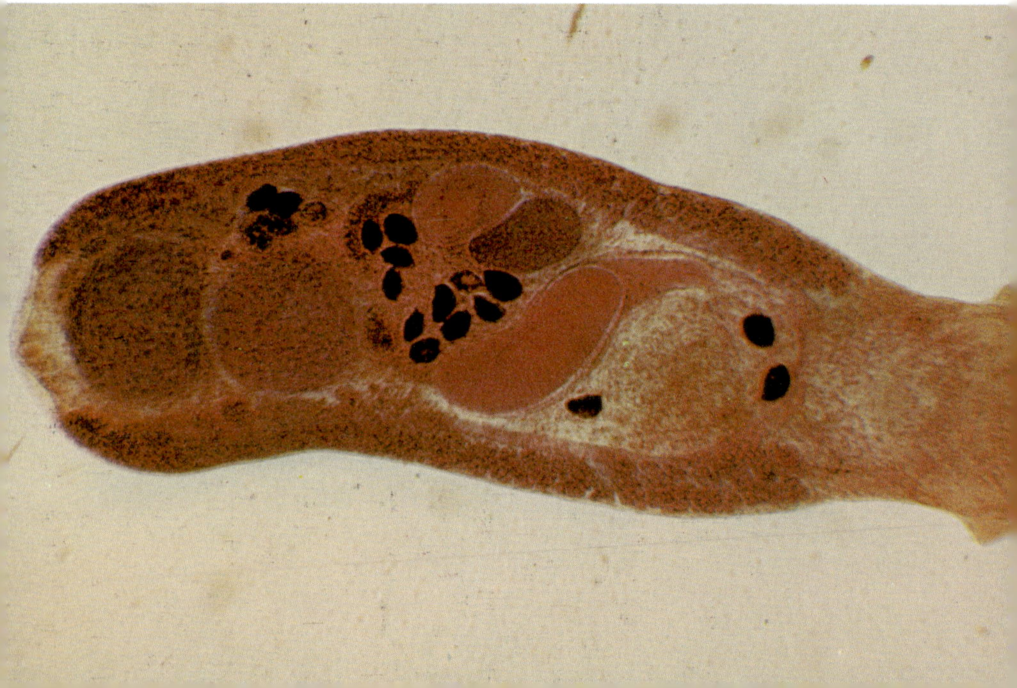

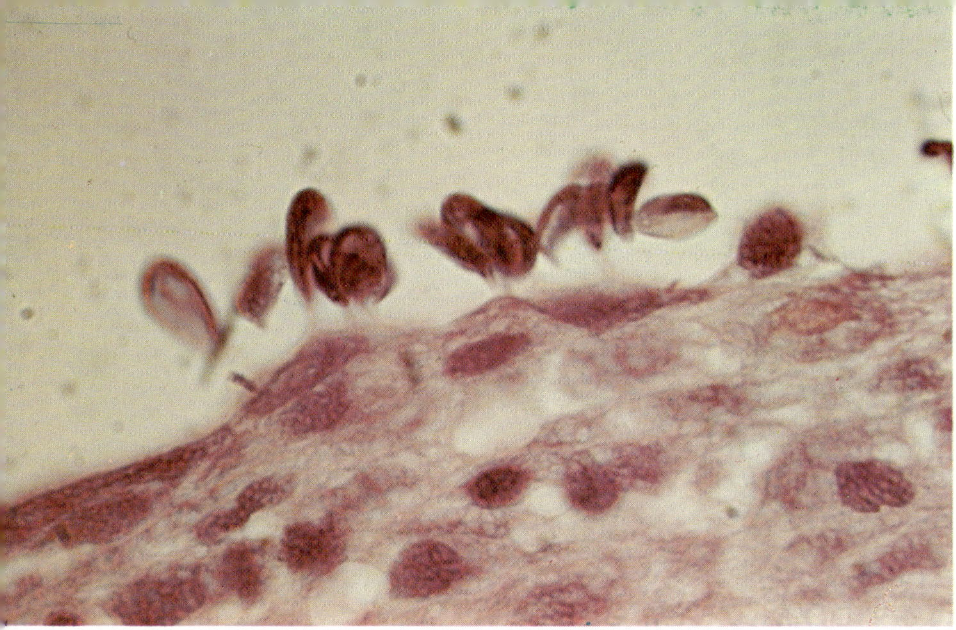

Costia attached to the skin of a trout.

One of the signs of costiasis is a "slime" on the skin of the host. Photo by Dr. G. Hoffman.

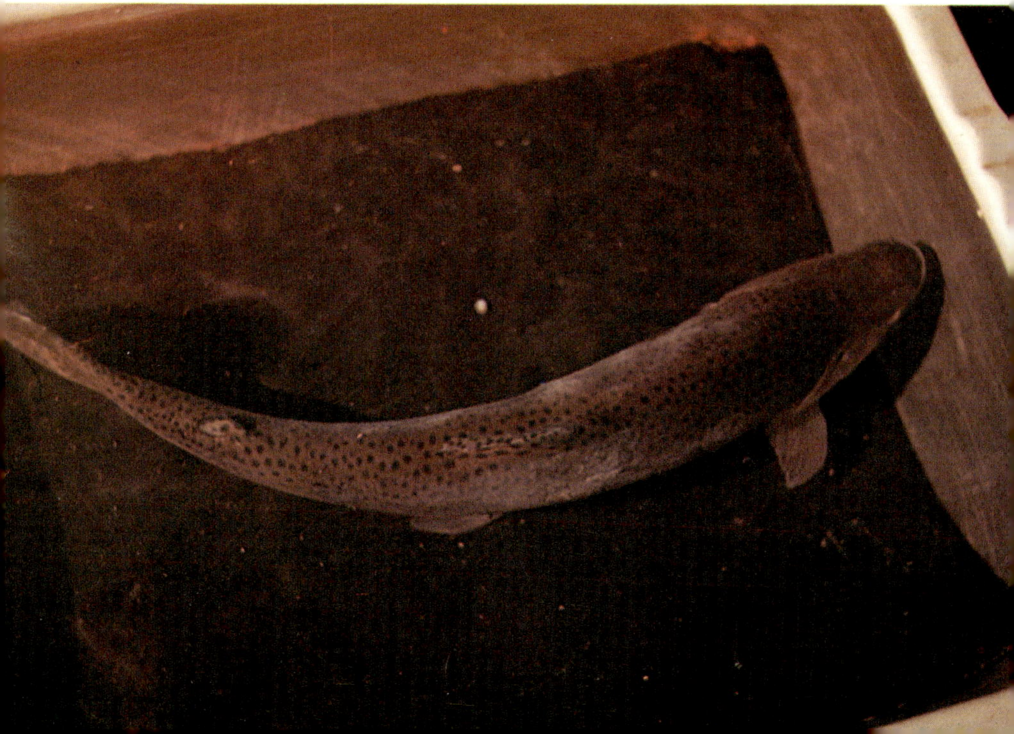

extreme cases they can quite easily be caught with the hand, as if they were "asleep." Concurrent with these characteristics, emaciation, sunken eyes and abnormal swimming movements will usually be observed. The gills look pale. The blood is found to contain elongate, biflagellate *Cryptobia.* A magnification of at least 300 times is essential for the investigation.

Incidence and prognosis: Since we do not tolerate fish leeches in the aquarium, the disease cannot spread there. Goldfish are occasionally affected. In wild catches of East African cichlids, this infection is fairly common. Treatment is unknown.

Trypanosoma

The blood of fish may be found to contain flagellates which closely resemble *Cryptobia* but possess only one flagellum. They belong to the genus *Trypanosoma.* So far, we do not know of a *Trypanosoma* species that constitutes a real danger to fish. Whether the organism concerned is a biflagellate, dangerous species of the

Trypanosoma elegans among red bloods cells of a gudgeon. The similarity to *Cryptobia* is obvious. Photo by Dr. Lom.

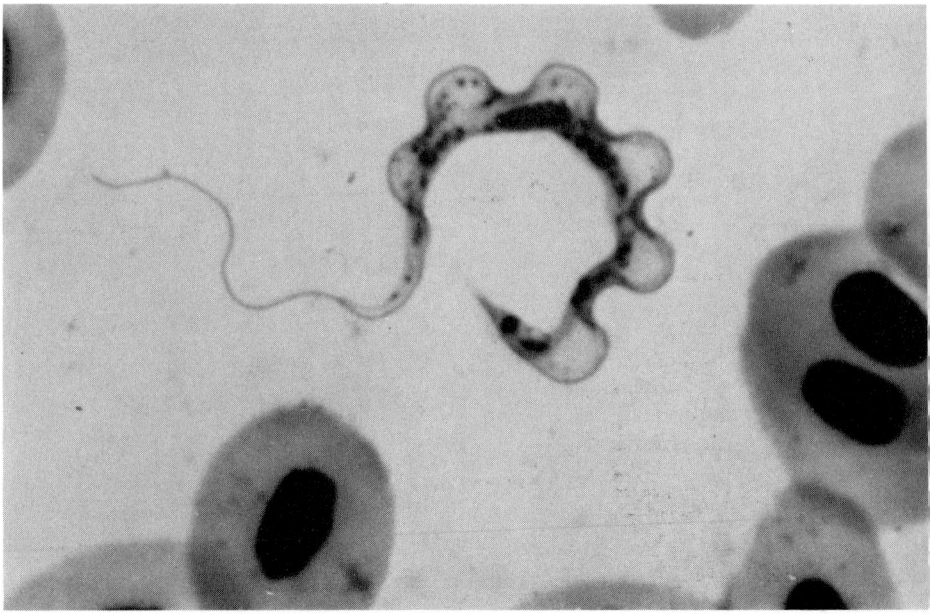

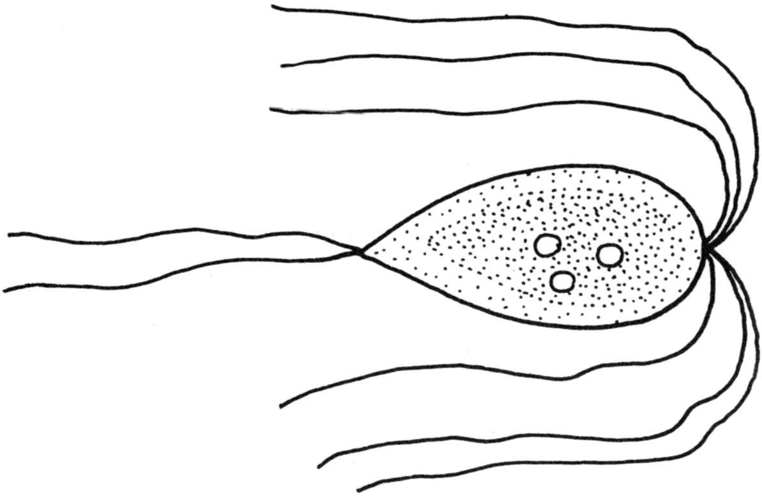

Hexamita has a more elongate body than the similar *Spironucleus*.

genus *Cryptobia* or a monoflagellate, harmless *Trypanosoma* can only be established by very close examination with a good microscope.

Hexamita

Etiology and diagnosis: Hexamita (obsolete name: *Octomitus)* is a minute flagellate with a length of approximately 7–13 microns. It seems to sway as it moves with its 6 anterior and 2 posterior flagella. *Hexamita* invades the gall bladder and occasionally the intestine. In severely affected animals the gall bladder becomes enlarged. In squash preparations the parasites are easy to detect.
Incidence and prognosis: Hexamita rarely occurs in ornamental fishes, but see *Spironucleus* for comparison.
Therapy: Preparations containing Metronidazol.

Spironucleus (PREVIOUSLY CLASSIFIED UNDER THE NAME *Hexamita)*

In the intestine of larger cichlids a certain flagellate measuring 8–13 microns (one micron equals 1/25,000 inch) in length is frequently found by the millions. In the intestine, this parasite is relatively harmless as a rule. It may, however, leave the intestine and migrate to other organs. This often results in death.

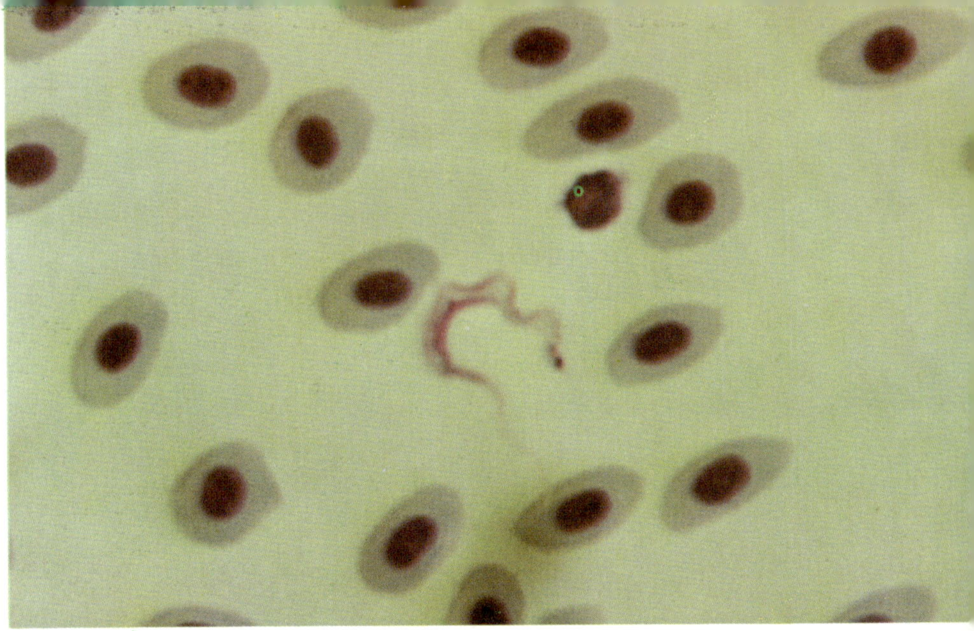

Trypanosoma is usually not dangerous to fishes in otherwise good health.

Differentiation of *Cryptobia* (below) and *Trypanosoma* is not easy without a good microscope. Photo by Dr. D. Becker.

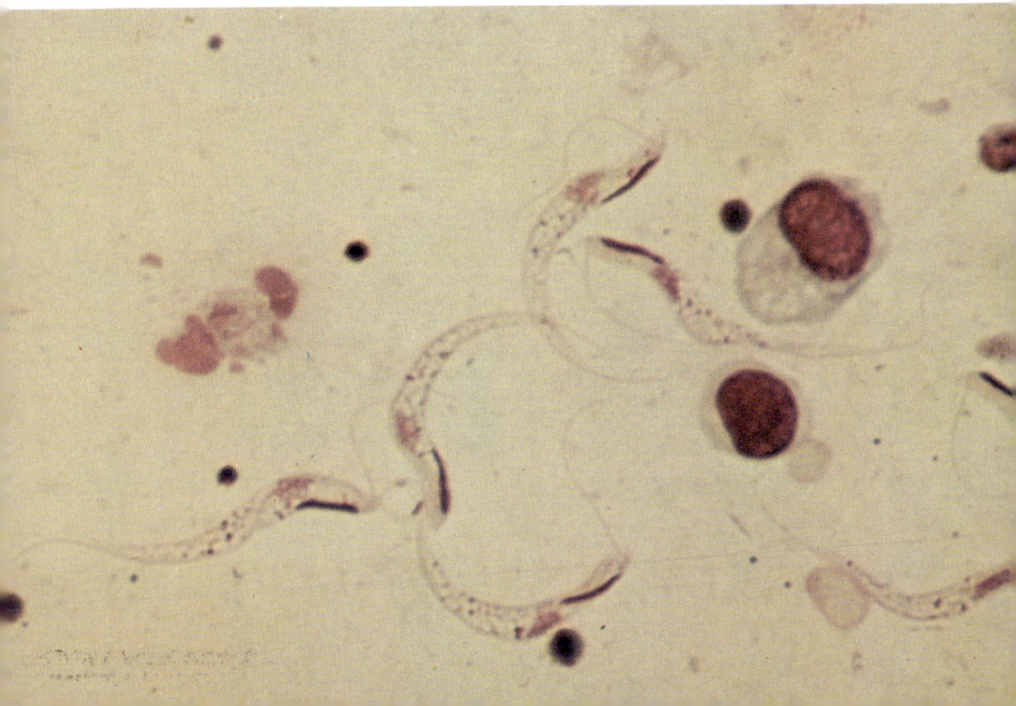

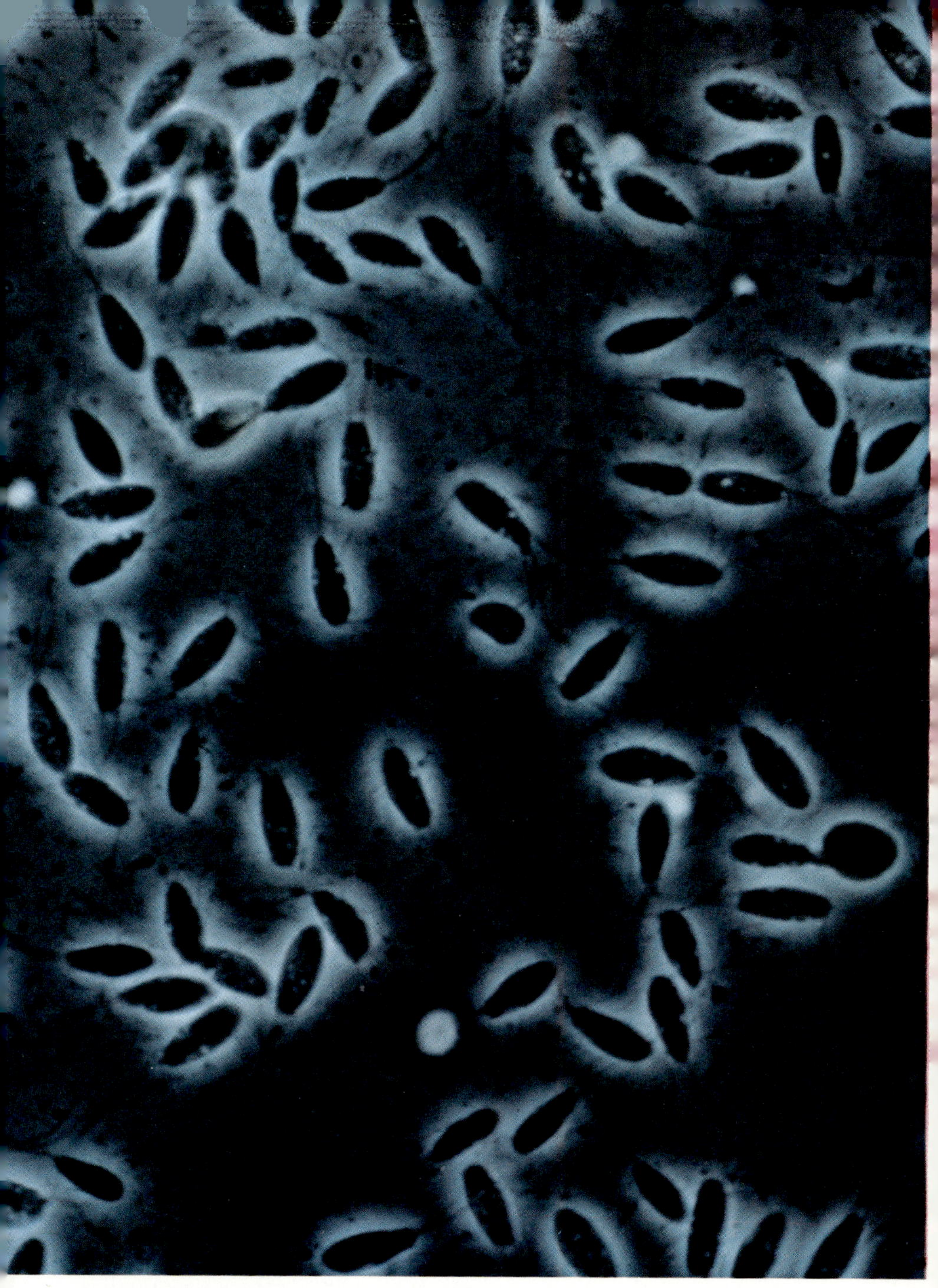

An intestinal smear from a fish heavily infected with *Hexamita*. Photo by Frickhinger.

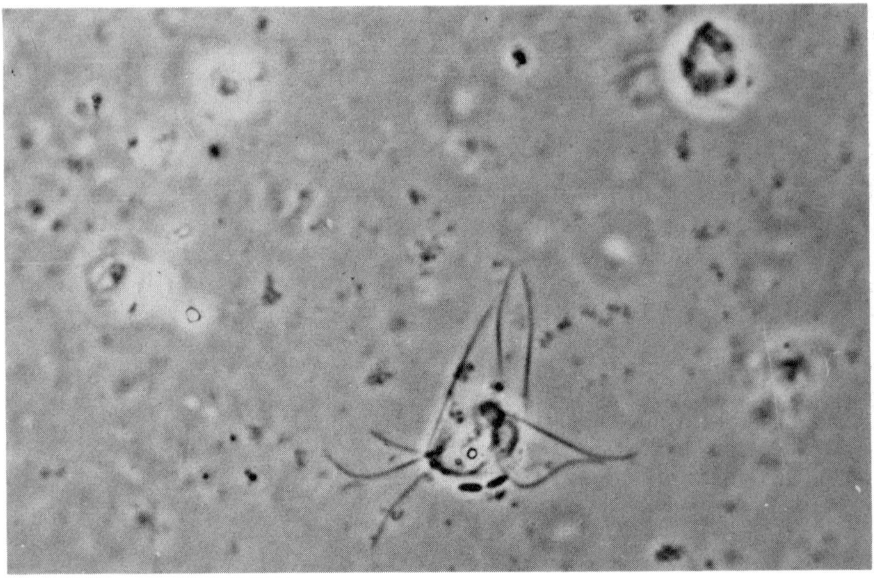

The flagellate *Spironucleus* from the gut of a discus. Notice the eight flagella. Photo by the author.

This gill from a discus which had died of *Spironucleus* infection is blocked by numerous small crystals. Photo by the author.

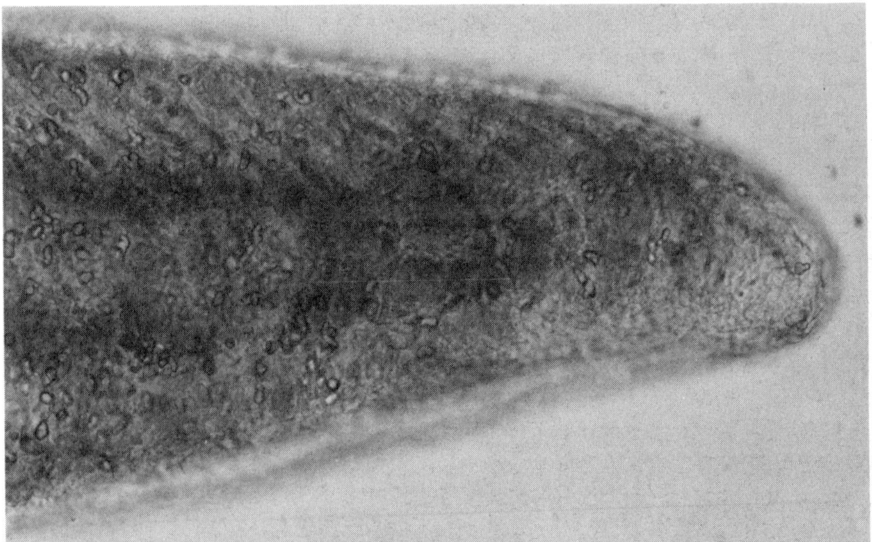

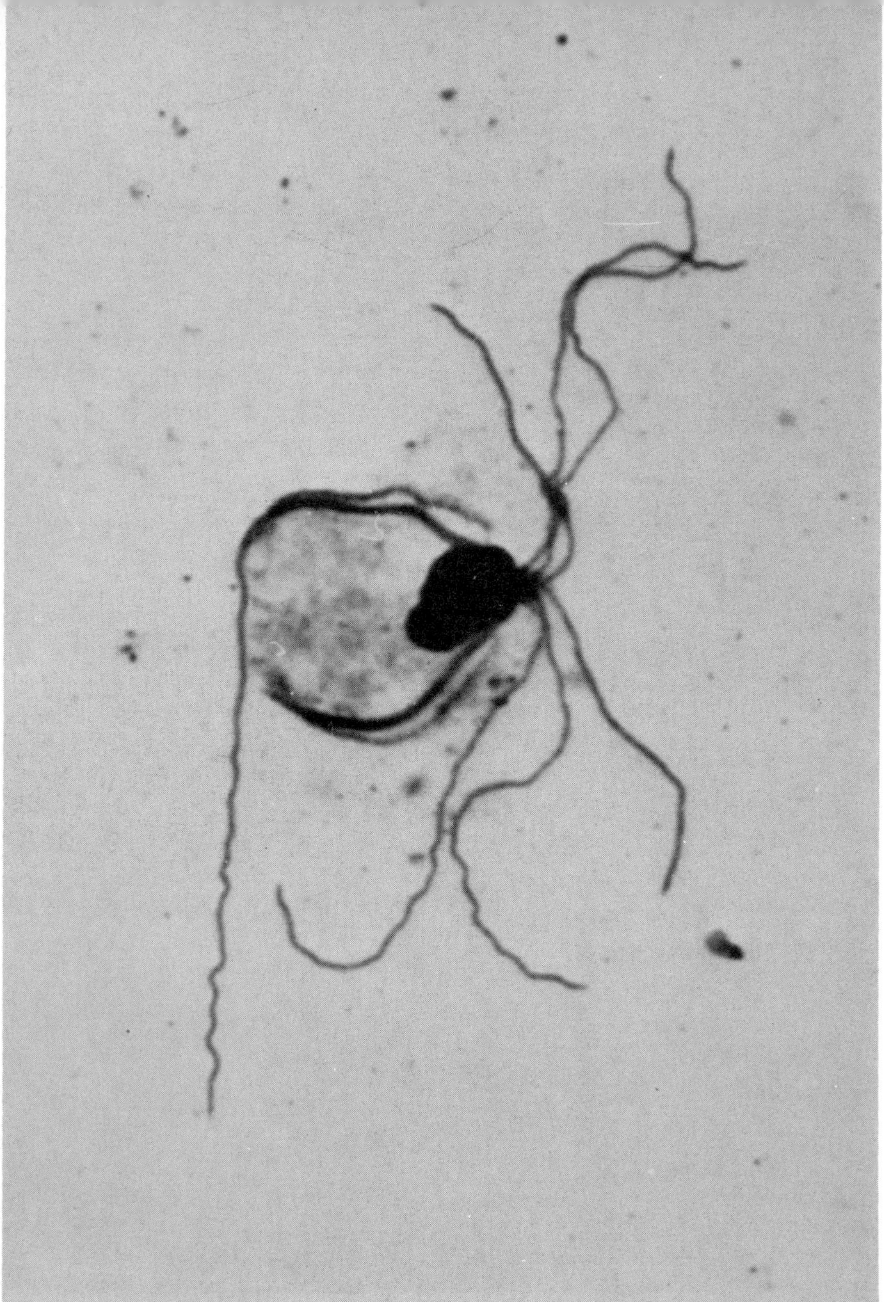

Spironucleus elegans, a parasite of frogs, is similar to the species found in discus. Photo by Dr. Lom.

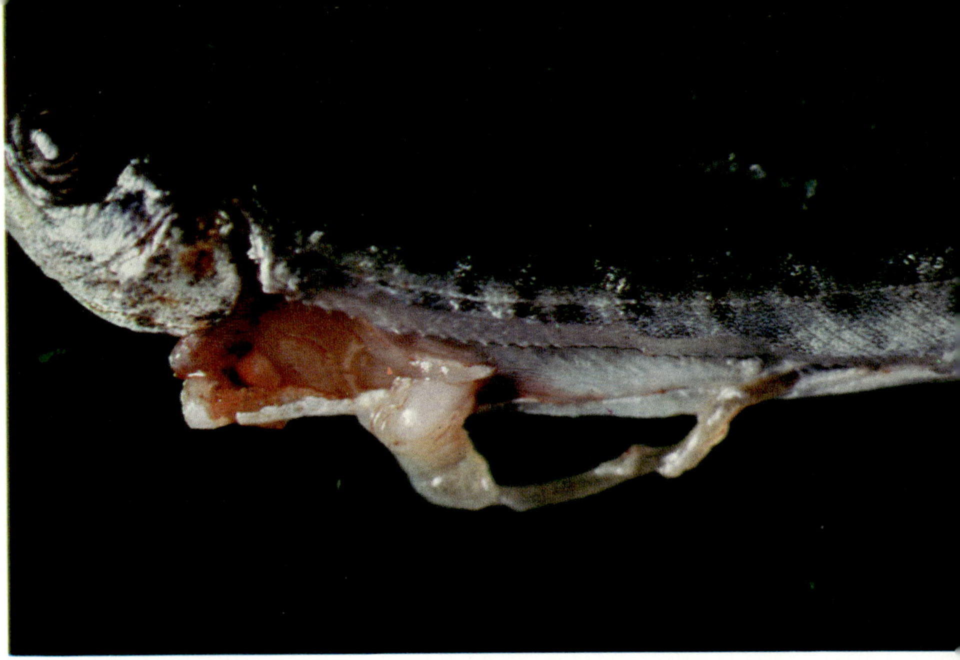

Hexamitiasis in a small trout. Notice the emaciated condition of the fish.

The adult cell of *Oodinium* lacks the flagella which are present in the immature. Photo by Dr. F. Meyer.

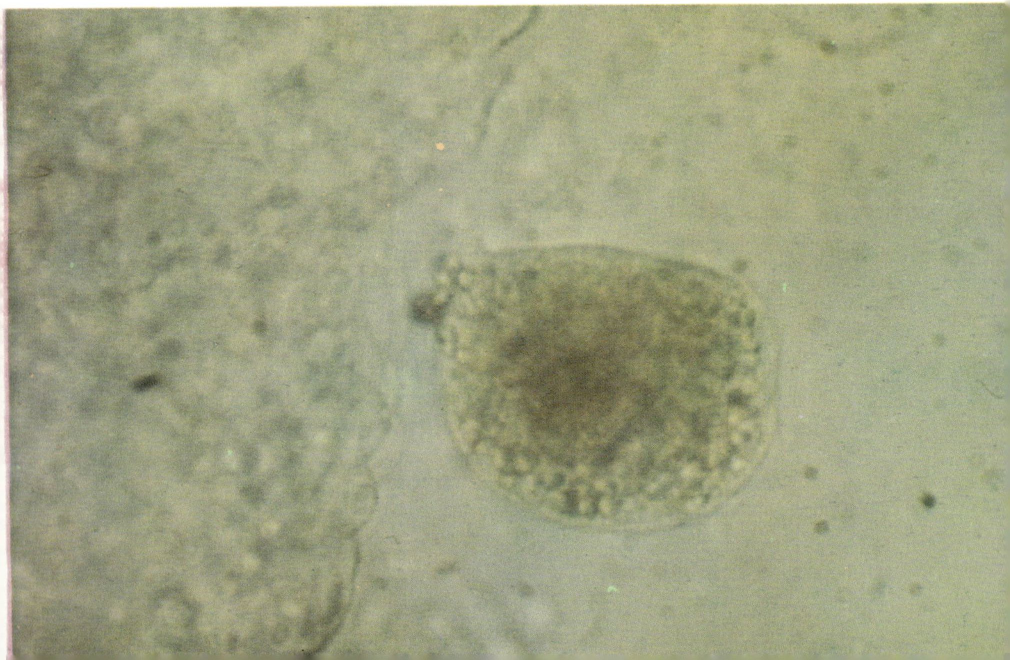

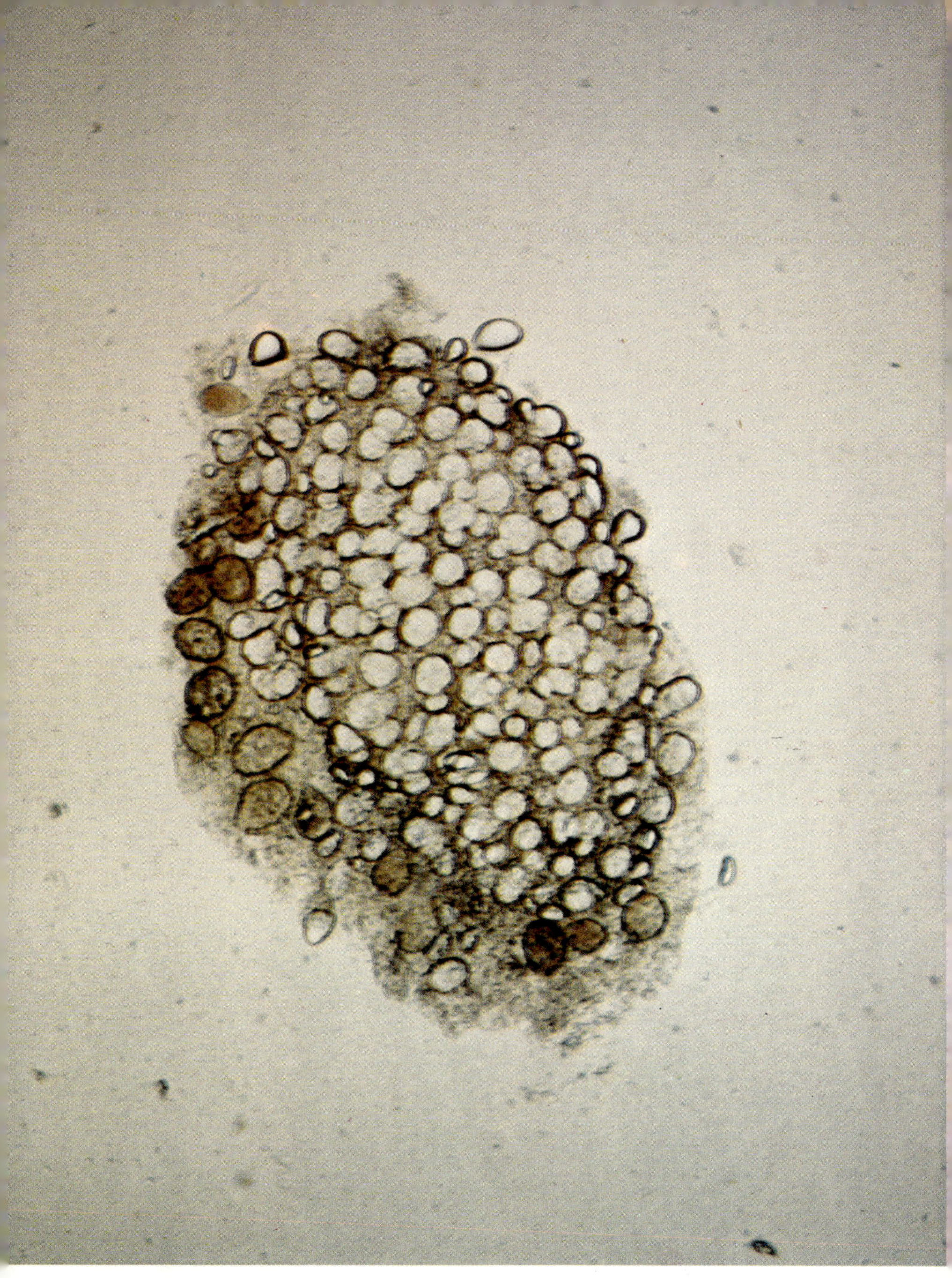

The reproduction of *Oodinium* through multiple divisions and flagellated swarmers allows it to rapidly reach high population densities. Photo by Frickhinger.

Clinical picture and diagnosis: Infected fish frequently show white, thread-like feces which adhere to the anus for a long time. An exact diagnosis can be made by examining freshly discharged feces or the intestinal content of a sacrificed animal under the microscope. The specimen will be teeming with highly motile flagellates which become apparent immediately.

Incidence and prognosis: The disease is common in angelfishes but does not seem to cause much suffering to them; discus and *Uaru*, on the other hand, frequently die of *Spironucleus* infections. African cichlids are, as a rule, quickly killed by this disease unless they are treated during the early stages. Whether the so-called "hole disease" of cichlids, causing the formation of small to fairly large holes in the head, is always due to *Spironucleus* infections is doubtful. "Hole disease" and these flagellates are, however, often found together. Control of the parasites is fairly easy. But once the internal organs, particularly the kidney, have suffered severe damage, treatment comes too late.

Therapy: Drugs containing Metronidazol are fairly effective. Metronidazol is found in certain tablets used in human medicine (ask your druggist), but drugs with this ingredient are now also being developed specifically for use in the aquarium and should be available in the near future. The administration of preparations based on antibiotics or mercury is less desirable.

Oodinium

Etiology: There are a variety of pathogenic *Oodinium* species, but the clinical picture is always more or less the same. All these species invade the epidermis and the gills and are sometimes found deeper within the host tissues as well. *Oodinium* may also parasitize the intestinal mucosa. The adult parasite has no flagella and cannot, at that stage, be identified as a flagellate. Having reached maturity, *Oodinium* drops off the fish and, at the bottom of the tank, becomes completely encased in a shell or test. Within this test, the organism undergoes division. Each daughter cell forms a new test and, within it, divides once more. This process is repeated several times until, during the final division, flagellated swarmers develop which in turn may attack fish.

Clinical picture and diagnosis: Infected fish show a white to dark coating. The signs of the disease may strongly remind one of those

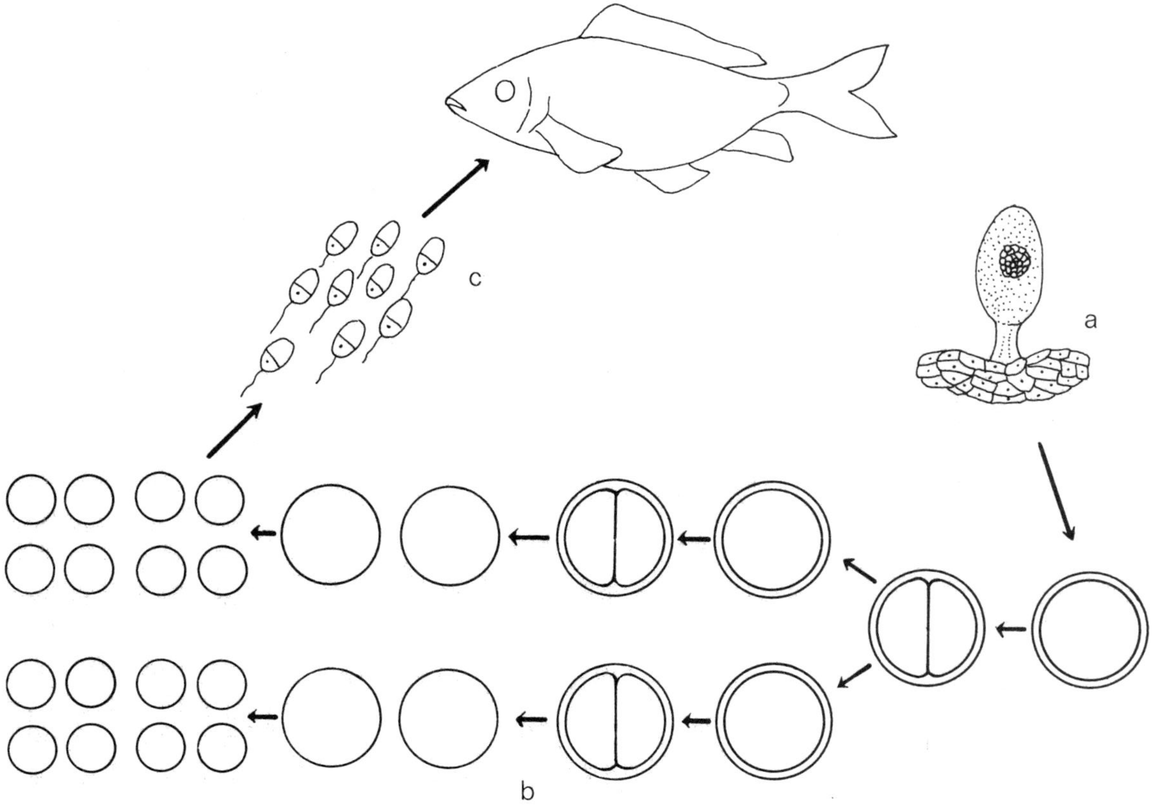

Life cycle of *Oodinium*: a, parasite on the skin of a fish; b, encystment and repeated division after dropping off host; c, flagellated swarmers infect fish.

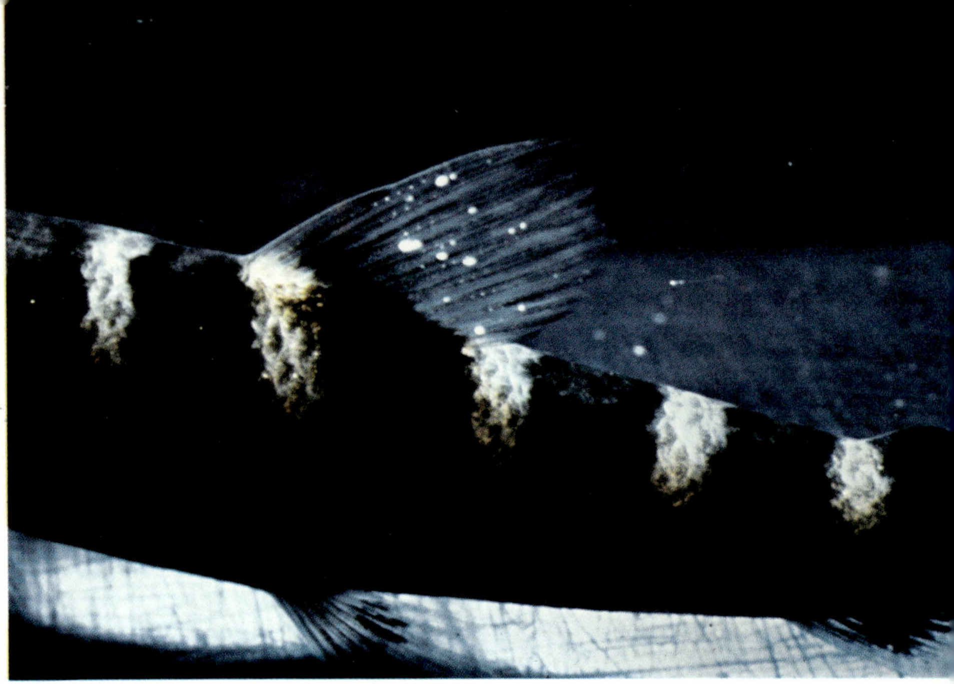

The spots caused by *Henneguya* resemble those of ich but under magnification lack large cells with curved nuclei. Photo by Frickhinger.

Cysts of *Henneguya* contain numerous spores with one or two long "tails." Photo by Dr. F. Meyer.

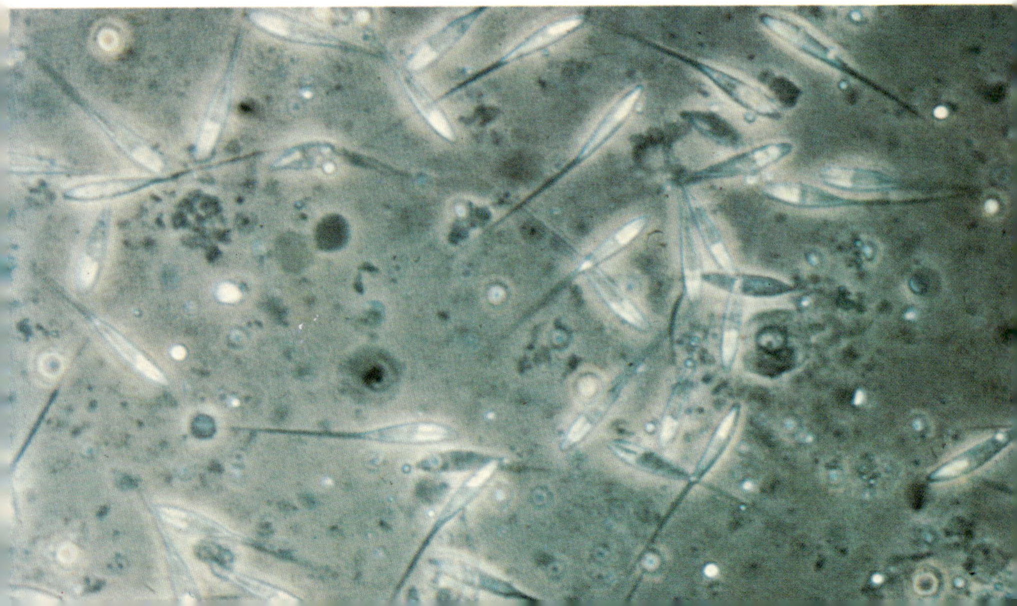

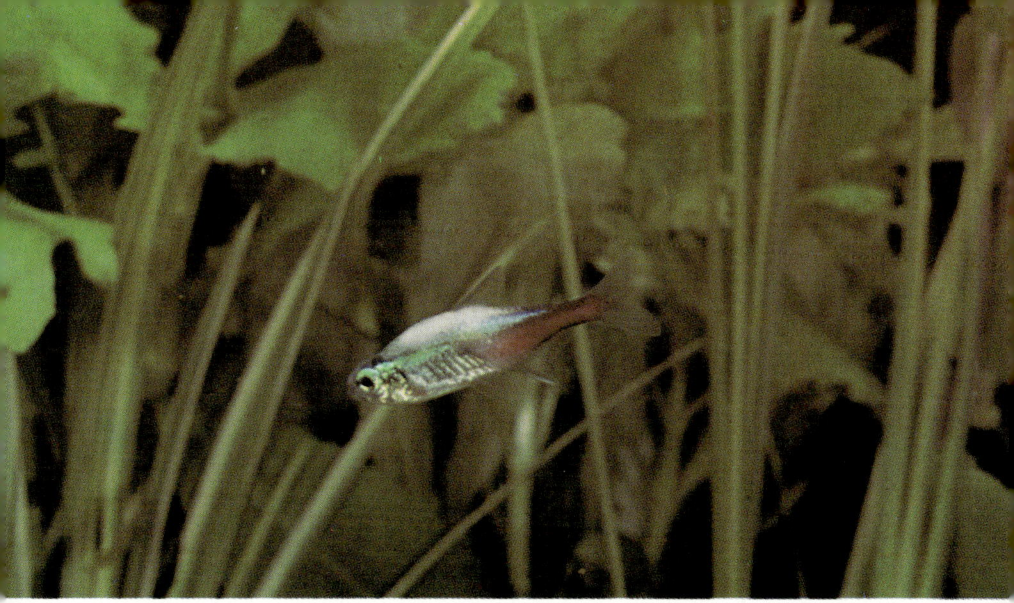

This neon tetra (*Paracheirodon innesi*) shows the characteristic white musculature of infection with *Plistophora hyphessobryconis*. Photo by R. Zukal.

Not all species of *Plistophora* occur in tetras. These are spores of *Plistophora ovariae* from the ovaries of the golden shiner. Photo by Dr. R. Summerfelt.

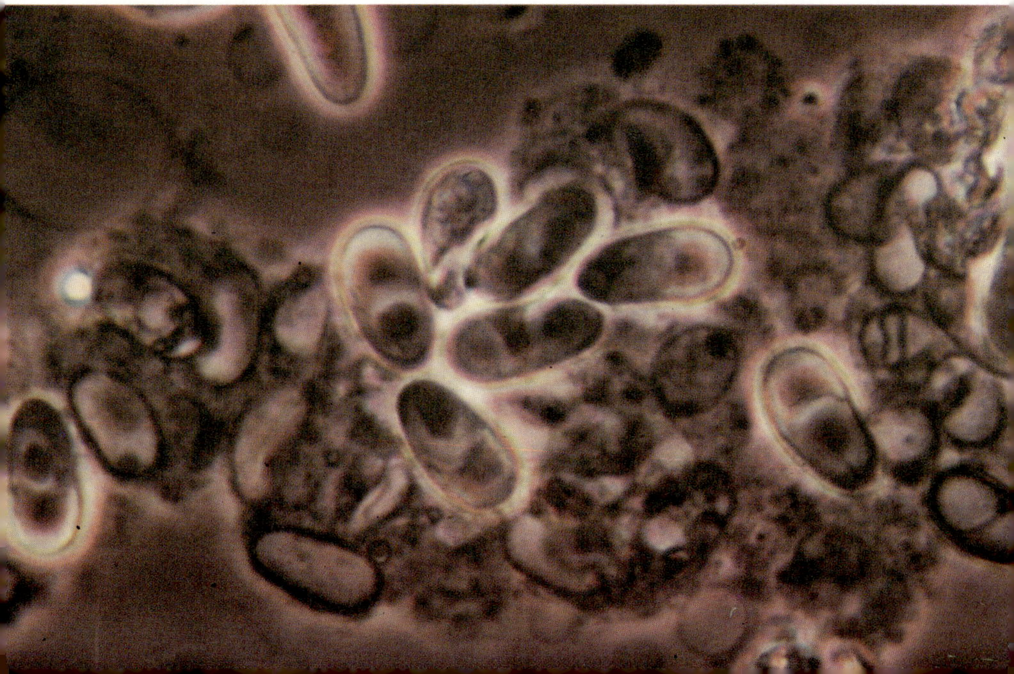

caused by *Ichthyophthirius*, except that the individual parasites (recognizable through the magnifying glass as tiny spots) are much smaller (20–70 microns). On the gills, too, the parasites can be seen as minute white specks. Under the microscope, *Oodinium* looks spherical to casket-like in shape and is usually seen to contain highly refractile granules. Finally, an intestinal smear should also be examined for parasites. Behavioral characteristics indicating an infection of the fish with *Oodinium* are scraping movements and, if the gills are intensely affected, difficulty in breathing and gasping for air.

Incidence and prognosis: Oodinium ocellatum is the causative agent of "coral fish disease" in salt water tanks. *Oodinium pillularis* and *Oodinium limneticum* (the latter known so far only from American tanks) cause "velvet disease" and can occur in most of our fresh-water aquarium fishes. The name "Colisa parasite," referring to its first appearance in gouramis, should therefore be avoided. The disease is often confused with *Ichthyophthirius*. A cure is possible, provided the disease is still in its early stages, but a relapse is not uncommon. If the disease remains untreated, it frequently drags on for a long time and usually ends in death.

Therapy: Oodinium is most effectively combated with long duration baths in copper sulfate. However, since the copper content of normal water, such as sea water, quickly diminishes, half the original dose should be added every third and fifth day. This may, however, result in an overdose. If the fish respond poorly, they have to be placed in fresh water immediately. Baths in chloromycetin or quinine often help too. Instead of copper, zinc may be added to the bath.

Sporozoa

All Sporozoa are parasites, and almost all of them have spores which form the resistant and infective stages. An immense variety of Sporozoa are known to be parasites of fishes living in their natural habitats, but so far only a few have been detected in aquaria (which need not necessarily mean that they do not occur there).

Plistophora hyphessobryconis

Etiology: The causative agent of the "neon tetra disease," *Plistophora hyphessobryconis* lives in the musculature of fish where it causes degeneration or even dissolution. The parasite forms spherical cysts (pansporoblasts), about 30 microns in size, which are frequently found in groups of up to 30. Within these pansporoblasts, spores of approximately 5 microns are formed. When the pansporoblast bursts the spores are released and expelled through the skin into the water. If a fish ingests such a spore with its food, a small amoeboid organism is liberated from it into the intestine. It penetrates the intestinal wall and enters the muscles where it then forms new pansporoblasts. The muscle is broken down in the process.

Clinical picture and diagnosis: Where the muscles have been destroyed whitish areas shine through the skin. This phenomenon is most marked in the neon, where the bright-green and also the red band may be interrupted by it. But the milky white zones that lie beneath the skin are conspicuous in other fishes, too. For the final diagnosis, a sample of affected muscle is teased and examined

Although *Plistophora hyphessobryconis* is usually thought of in connection with the neon tetra, it also occurs in other species of fish. However, it is not known to occur in the cardinal tetra (*Cheirodon axelrodi*). Photo by R. Zukal.

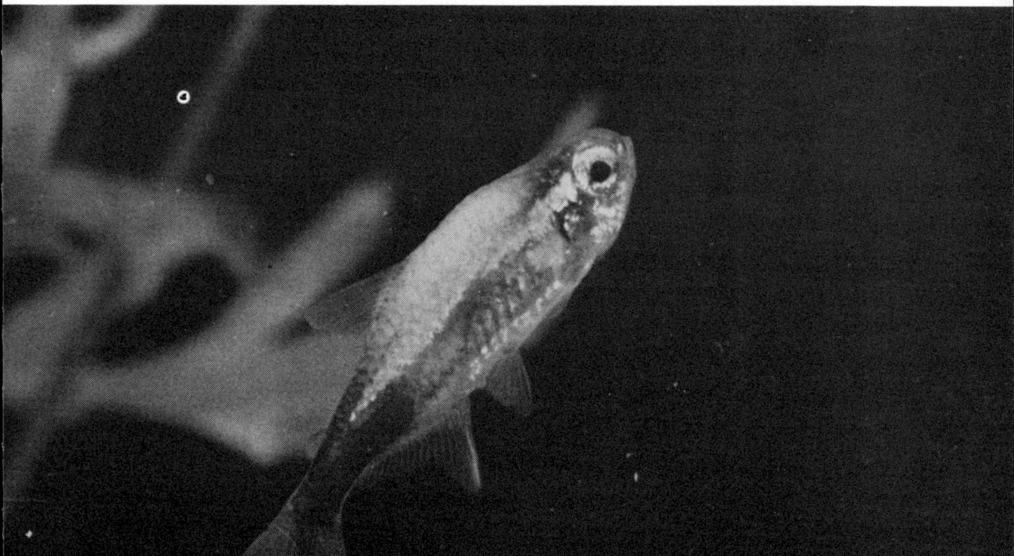

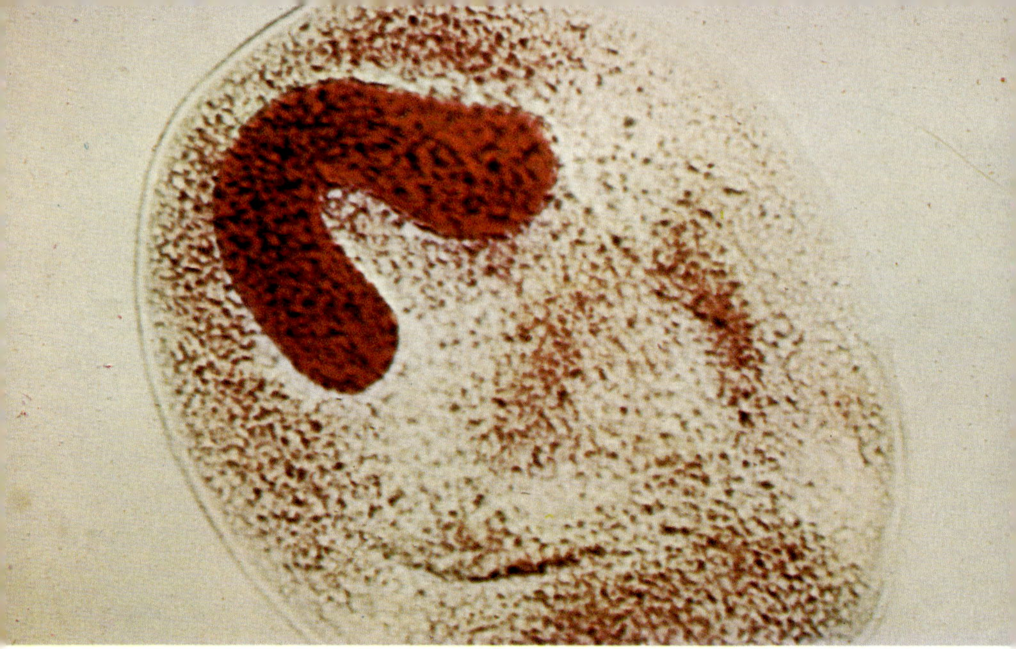

The mature cell of *Ichthyophthirius multifilis* is easily recognized by its large, horseshoe-shaped nucleus. Photo by Dr. F. Meyer.

If caught in the early stages where just a few spots are visible, as in the fins of this platy (*Xiphophorus maculatus*), ich can be relatively easy to cure. Photo by M.F. Roberts.

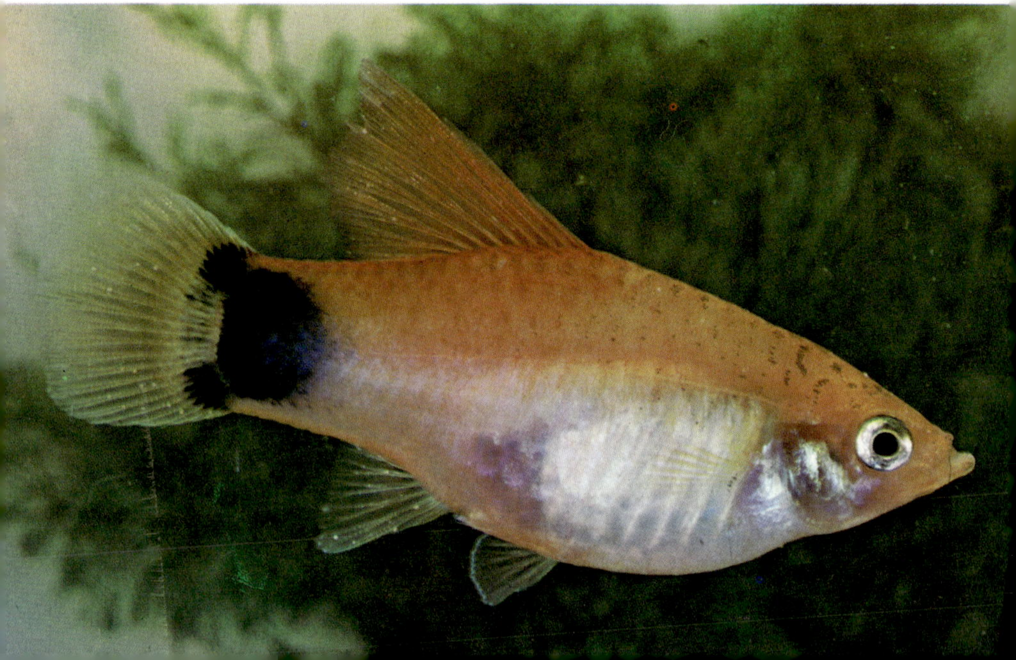

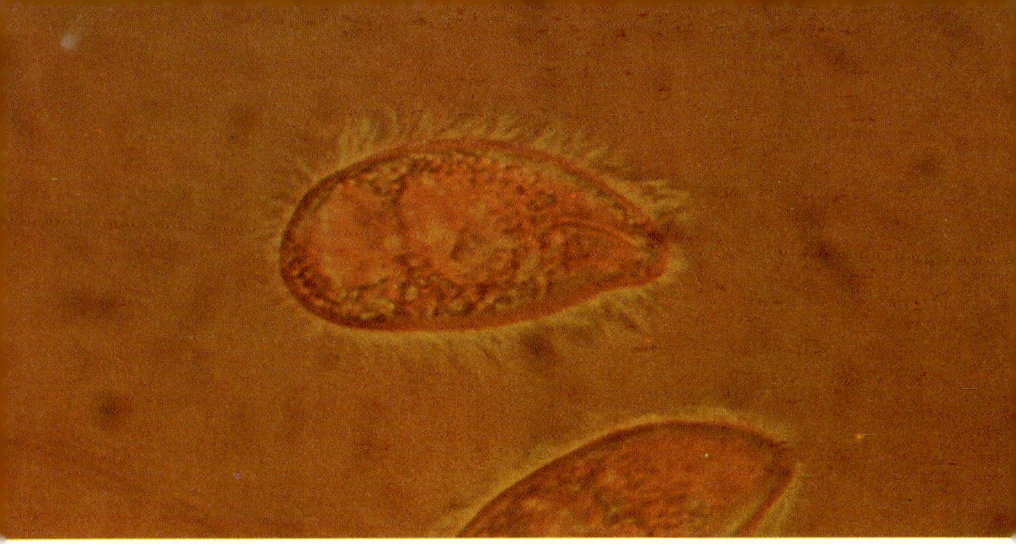

Cryptocaryon irritans, the cause of salt water ich, also goes through a free-swimming swarmer stage like that of freshwater ich. Unfortunately it is harder to treat than the usual ich. Photo by Drs. F.R. Nigrelli and G.D. Ruggieri, Osborne Lab., New York Aquarium.

Infections of salt water ich are often heavier and more deadly than those of freshwater ich. Photo by Frickhinger.

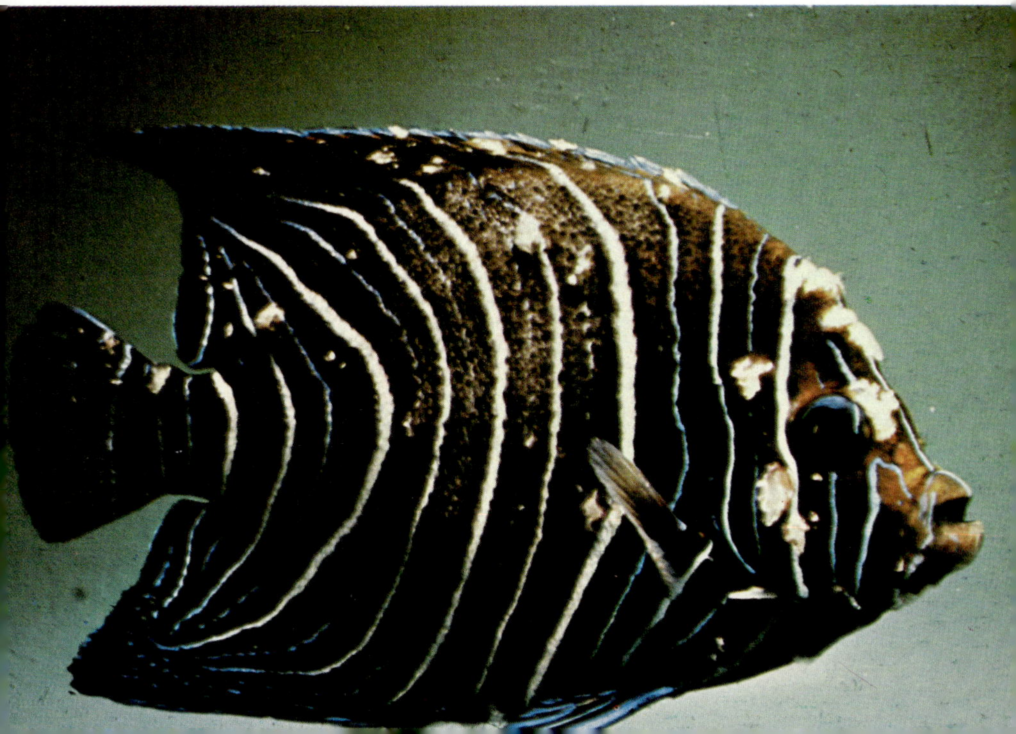

under the microscope. At a magnification of 150 times, the spherical, considerably refractile (and hence dark-looking) pansporoblasts are very obvious.

Incidence and diagnosis: Contrary to the name "neon tetra disease," *Plistophora* does not confine itself to *Paracheirodon innesi* but attacks most characins. The disease has also been observed in *Brachydanio rerio.* It is very likely that yet other fishes can contract it, too. The cardinal tetra *(Cheirodon axelrodi)* is not susceptible to it.

Therapy and prophylaxis: Effective drug treatment is not known. All assertions of a cure having been found for the disease have so far proved mistaken. It is possible, however, to prevent renewed infection in diseased stock by keeping the animals above a fine and closely perforated bottom plate or netting. The water underneath the bottom plate or network is siphoned off with a powerful filter (operated by a rotary pump) and poured over a very tightly packed layer of nylon wool. Then the fish cannot become reinfected. Severely affected specimens will die and should be removed immediately; the rest will recover.

The spores of *Plistophora hyphessobryconis* are quite distinctive. Photo by Dr. Lom.

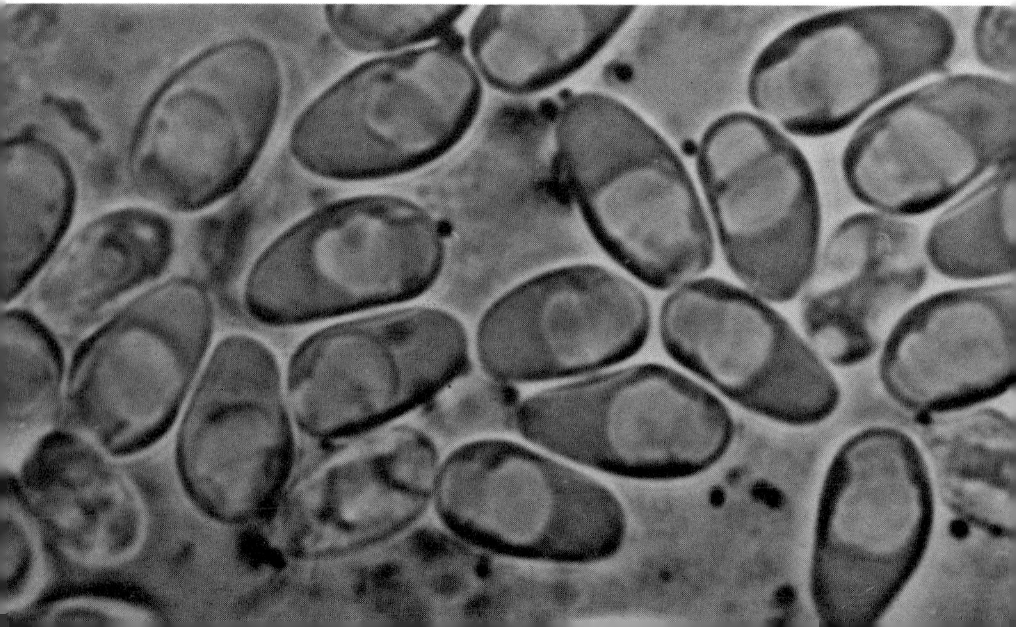

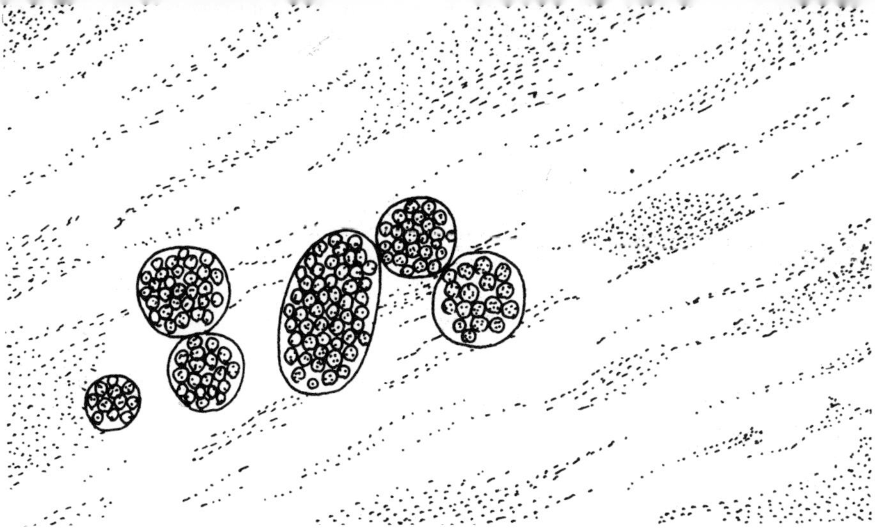

The pansporoblasts of *Plistophora* occur in large numbers within what look like small sacks of thin membrane. Each pansporoblast contains many spores. Photo below by R. Geisler.

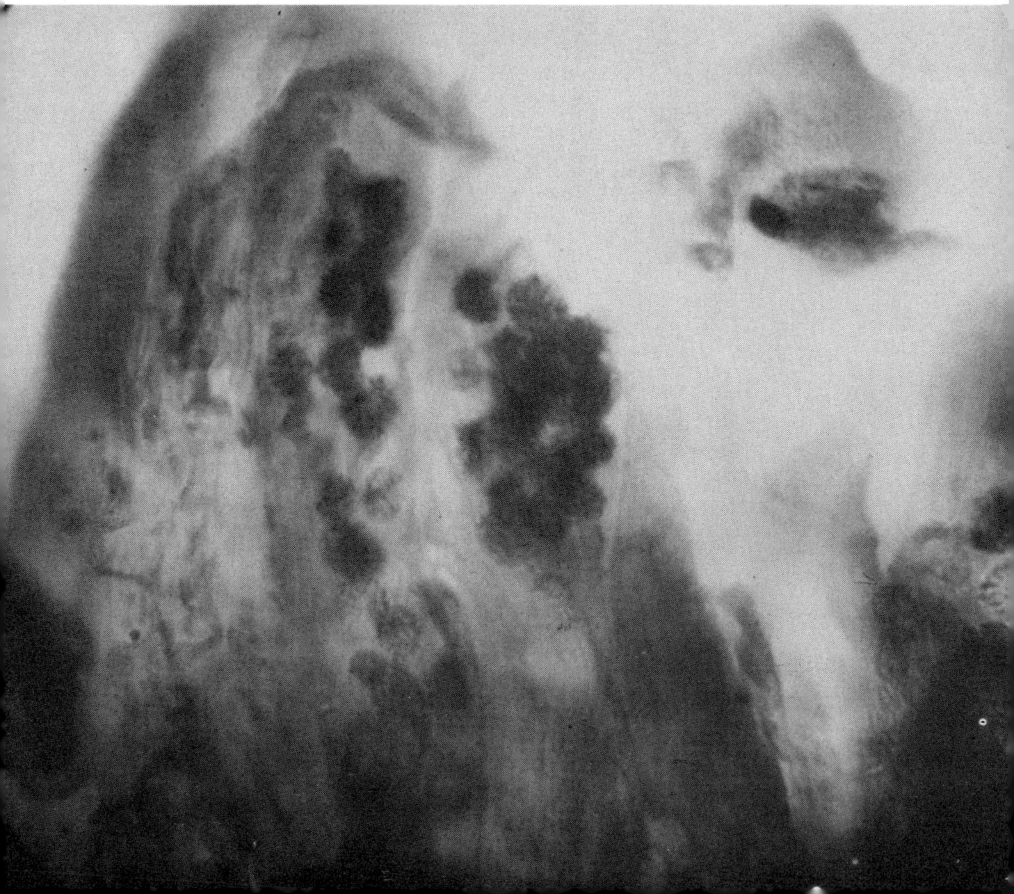

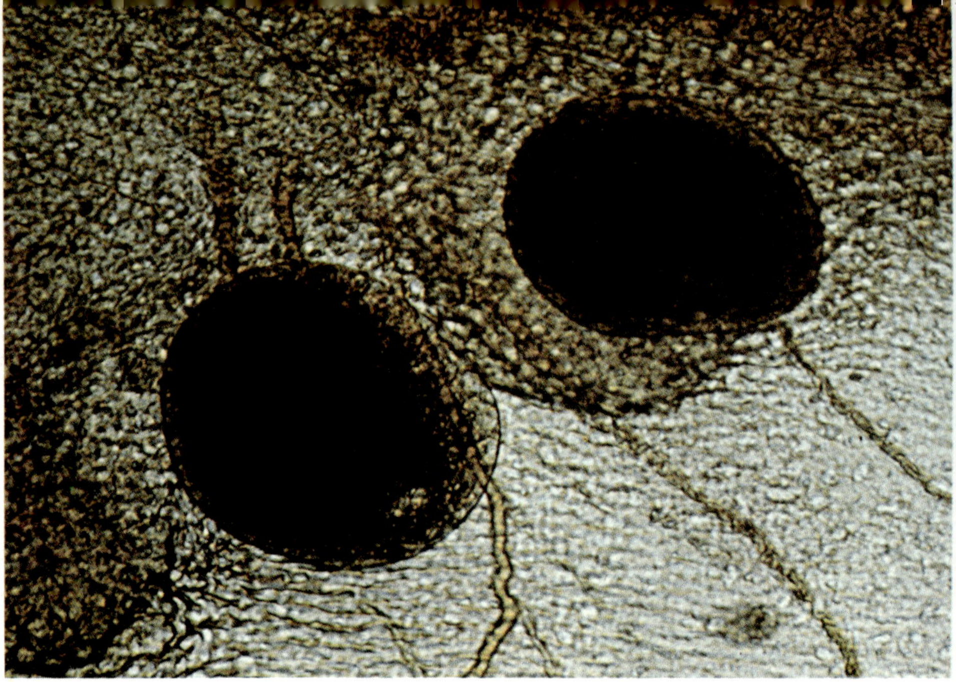

The mature cells of *Cryptocaryon irritans* are very similar to those of *Ichthyophthirius multifilis*. Photo by Frickhinger.

The gill parasite *Trichodina* is a scourge of commercial fish and also a nuisance in the aquarium. Photo by Dr. F. Meyer.

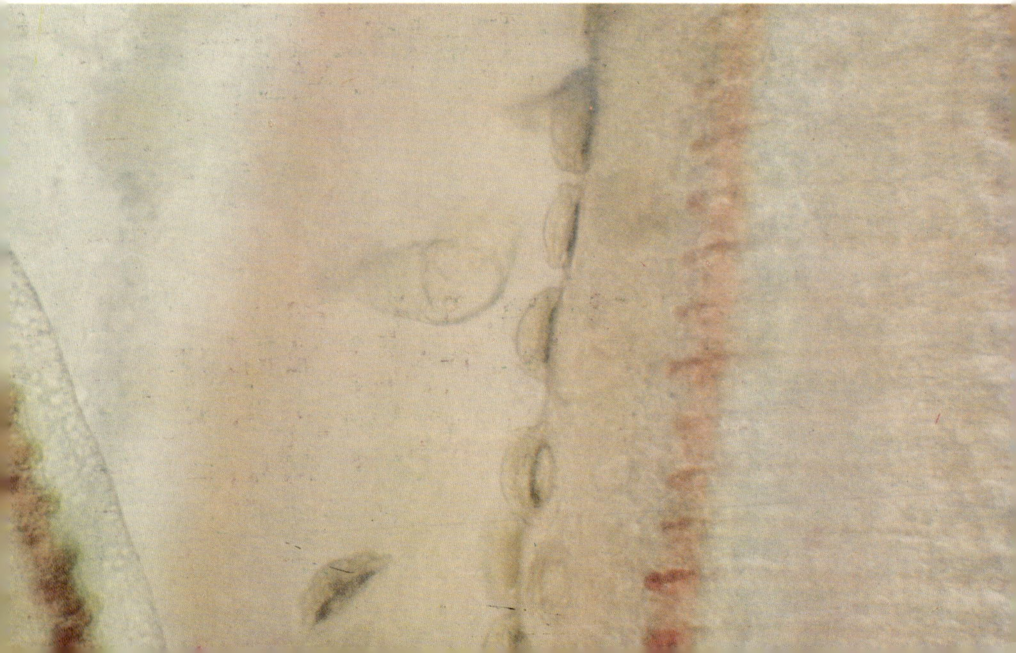

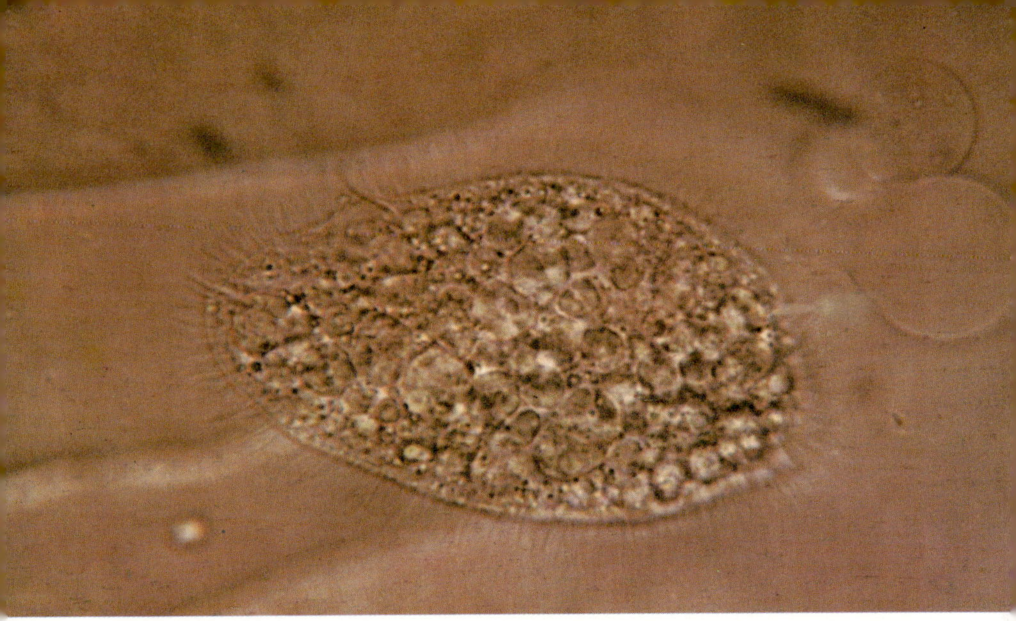

The pear-shaped *Tetrahymena corlissi* has recently been found to be very dangerous to guppies and has been dubbed the "guppy killer." Photo by Dr. J. Camper.

Ambiphrya (formerly called *Scyphidia*) can occur in large numbers on the fins of fishes. Their shape is usually distinctive. Photo by Dr. F. Meyer.

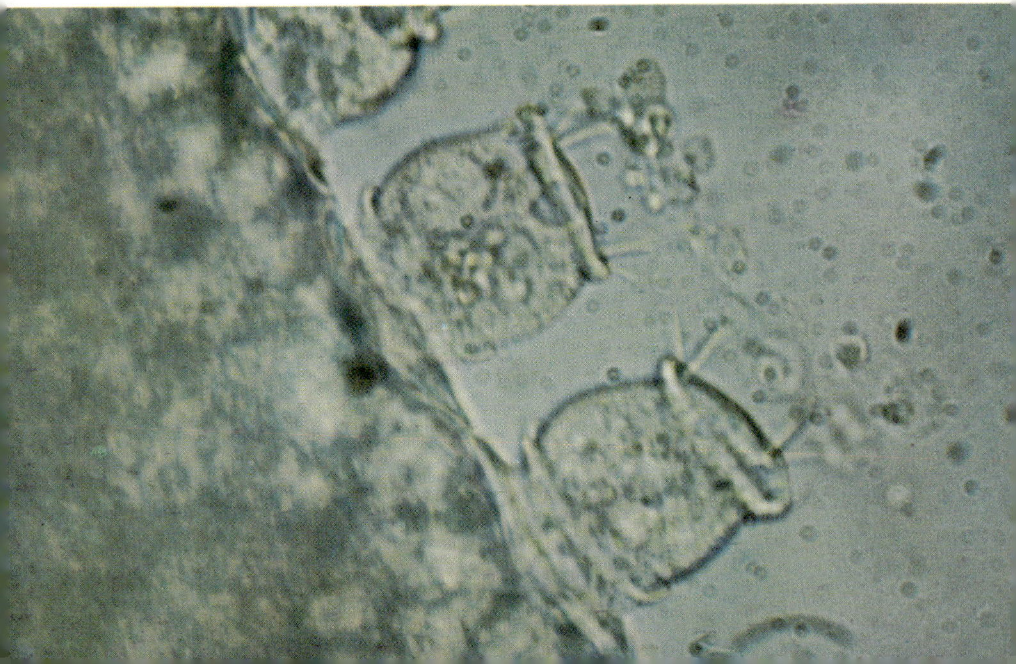

NODULAR DISEASES CAUSED BY SPOROZOANS

A number of sporozoans form small nodules in the internal organs, on the gills or on the skin of fish, which contain masses of spores that can infect other fish. Fishes living in their natural habitat are affected by a great variety of such parasites. In freshwater aquarium fishes, these sporozoans have only been found occasionally, usually in wild catches. To what extent salt water tanks are affected has so far not been established.

Clinical picture and diagnosis: The clinical picture varies very considerably, depending on the organs that have been infected. The nodules may be microscopically small up to the size of a pinhead. In squash preparations under the microscope the spores appear as single cells which are not interconnected, but to discern them we need to use powerful objectives. Many spores will be found to have 1 to 4 conspicuous, highly refractile bodies, the polar capsules. Certain species may form nodules on the fins which can be confused with *Lymphocystis*, but in a true *Lymphocystis* infection no spores are present.

Anyone seeing the white spots on the fin of this *Ctenopoma* would suspect ich. Yet the condition failed to respond to the usual ich cures. Photo by the author.

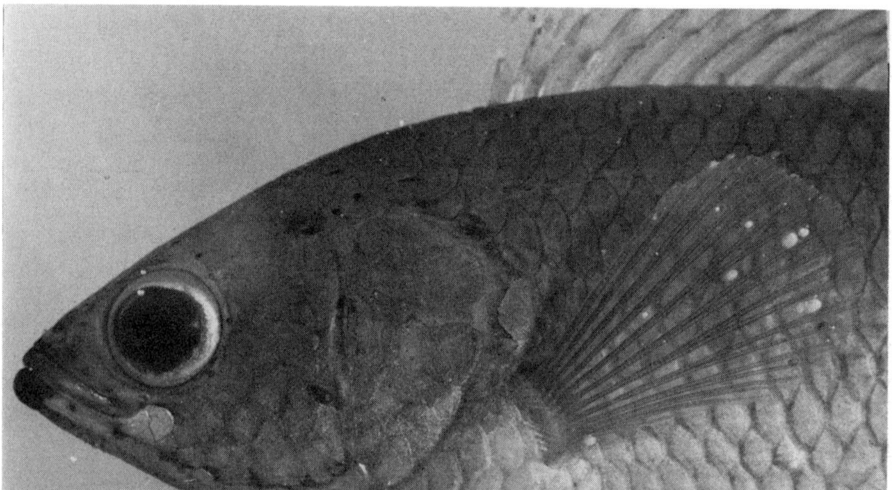

Closer examination of the white spots revealed them to be the cysts of *Henneguya pinnae*, a sporozoan which does not have a life cycle like that of ich. Photo by the author.

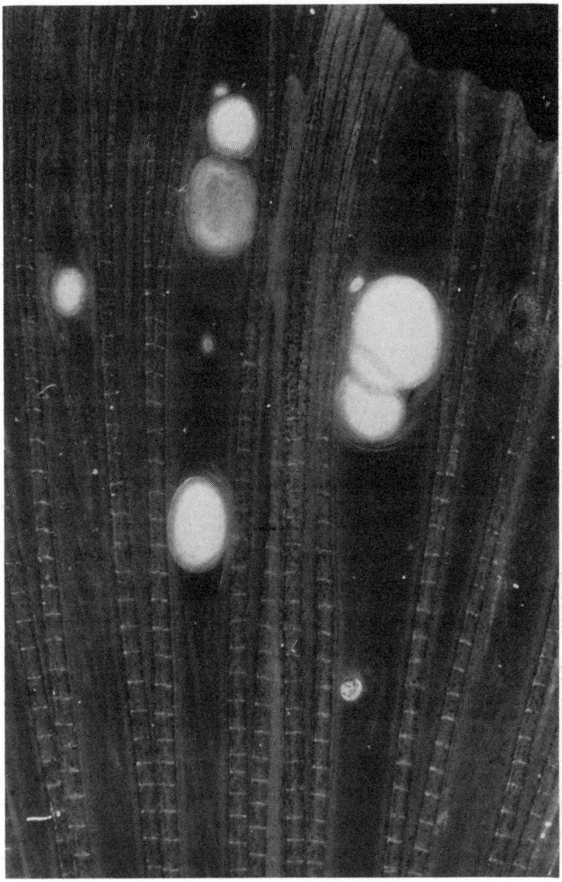

Incidence and prognosis: Sporozoans can occur in all species of ornamental fishes. Infections usually enter the tanks with wild catches or imports from East Asian hatcheries. However, with the exception of *Plistophora*, these infections do not usually last in our aquaria.

Therapy and prophylaxis: Where internal organs and the gills are affected, treatment is not possible. Diseased fishes have to be removed. Nodules confined to the outer areas of the fins may be cut off, but this method of treatment is not worth attempting unless the fish concerned are very valuable specimens, since there is great danger that very minute nodules are being overlooked. Even in a case like this, it is always better to kill the infected animals. The tanks also have to be disinfected.

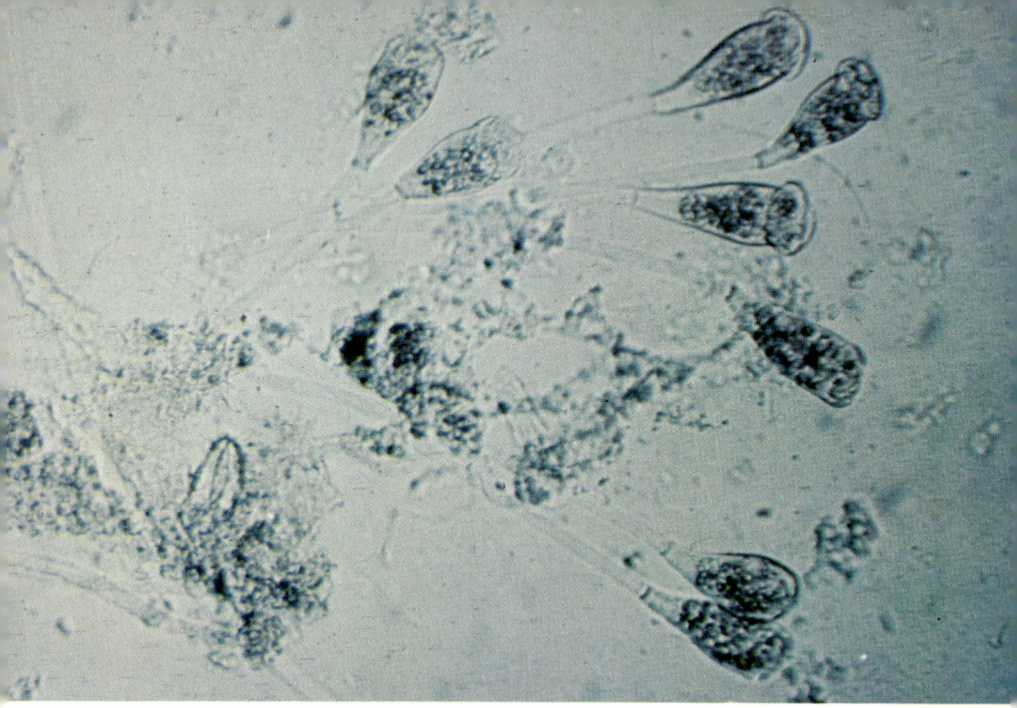

The stalked protozoans such as *Epistylis* are seldom a great nuisance either in the aquarium or in the wild. Occasionally, however, they can form large colonies on the skin of fishes, such as the warmouth bass below, and cause minor damage. Photos by Dr. W. Rogers.

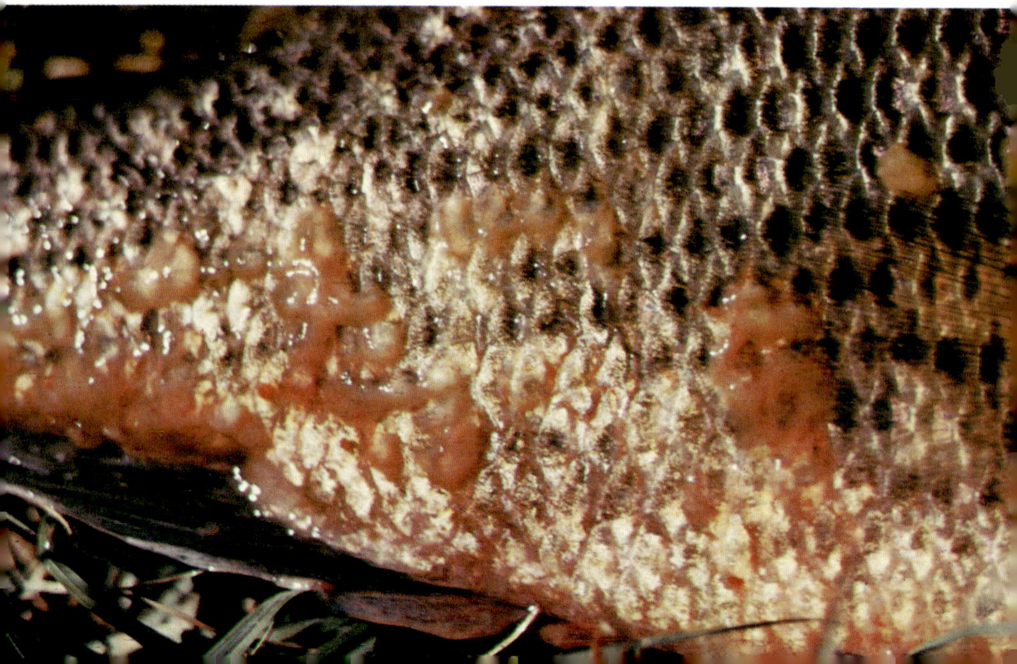

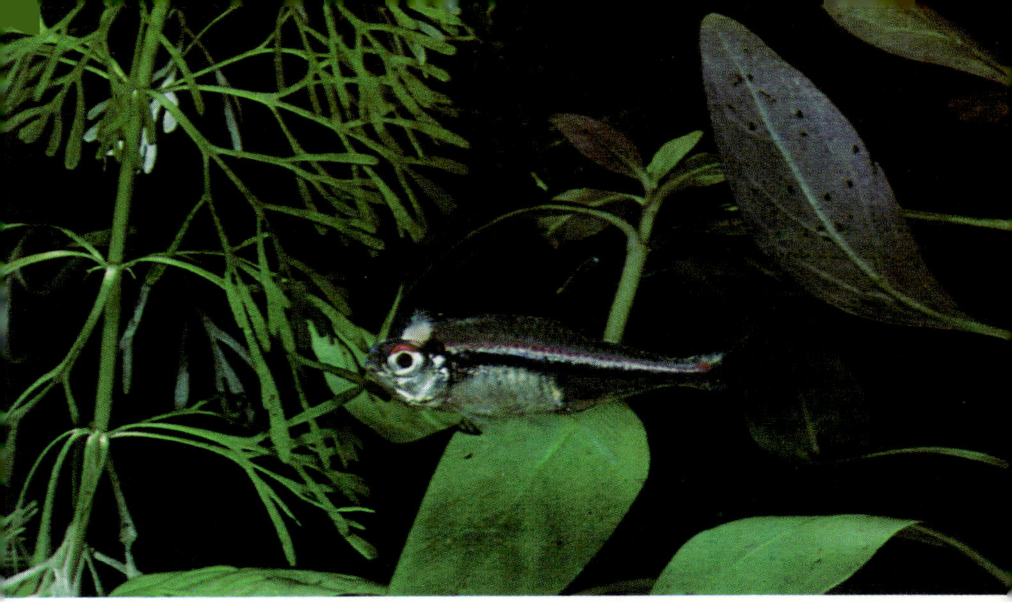

Although fungus infections can occur on almost any part of the fish, they are more common on the fins. This tetra probably lost a few scales behind the head during handling, thus opening a path for the infection. Photo by R. Zukal.

A close up view of *Saprolegnia* shows it to consist of numerous ramifying filaments. Photo by Dr. D. McDaniel.

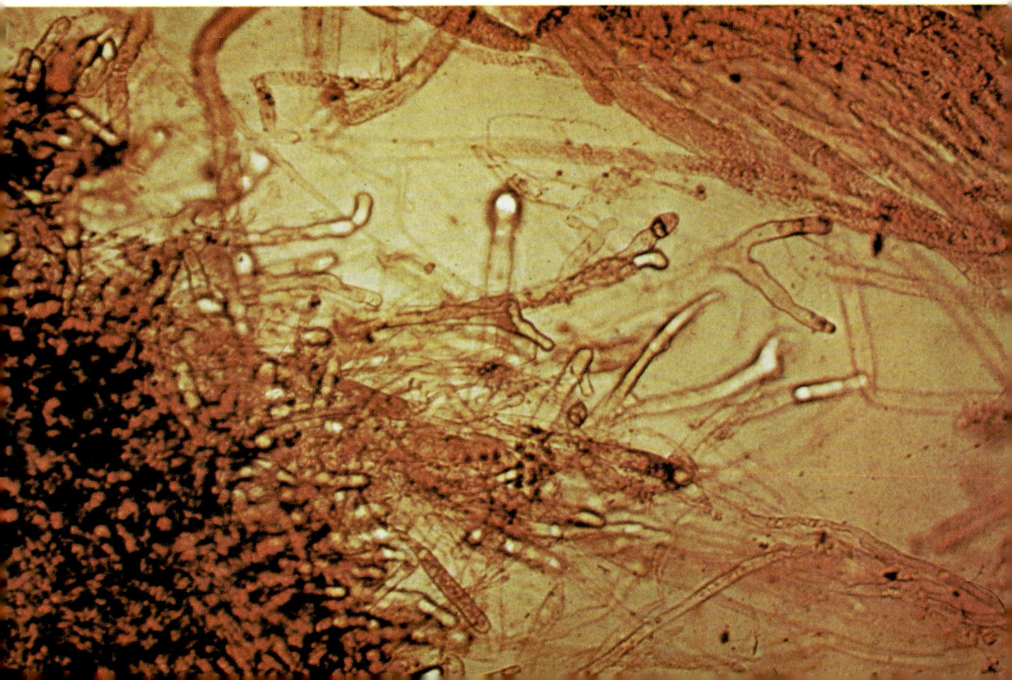

The ciliates, one of which, the slipper animalcule, is familiar to us as a food for fry, are unicellular organisms whose surface is completely or partially covered with cilia. Characteristically, they possess a large vegetative nucleus (macronucleus) which is responsible for metabolic processes and a small generative nucleus (micronucleus) concerned with sexual reproduction.

Ichthyophthirius multifilis

Etiology: Ichthyophthirius is a large ciliate visible to the naked eye. Its size, up to 1 mm, varies according to the size of the infected fish and external circumstances. It is spherical in shape and the cilia are evenly distributed over the whole surface. The large, horseshoe-shaped macronucleus is usually quite obvious. Another characteristic is its constant rotating movement.

The fully grown parasite drops off the host, surrounds itself with a capsule and fixes itself onto a plant or a stone. Capsules which for some reason or another fail to attach themselves to a solid object do not usually develop any further. Inside the capsule the parasite undergoes division until eventually 250 to 1,000 small (about 30 microns in size), pear-shaped, ciliated swarmers have been produced. The capsule bursts and the swarmers swim off to attach themselves anywhere on the surface of a fish, though caudal

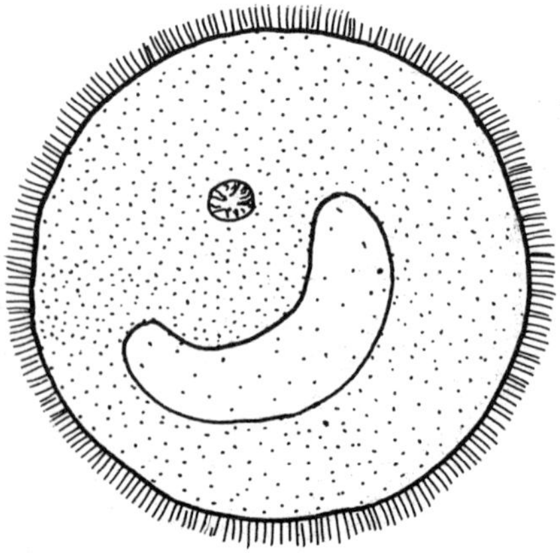

The shape and size of the nucleus are enough to identify *Ichthyophthirius multifilis*.

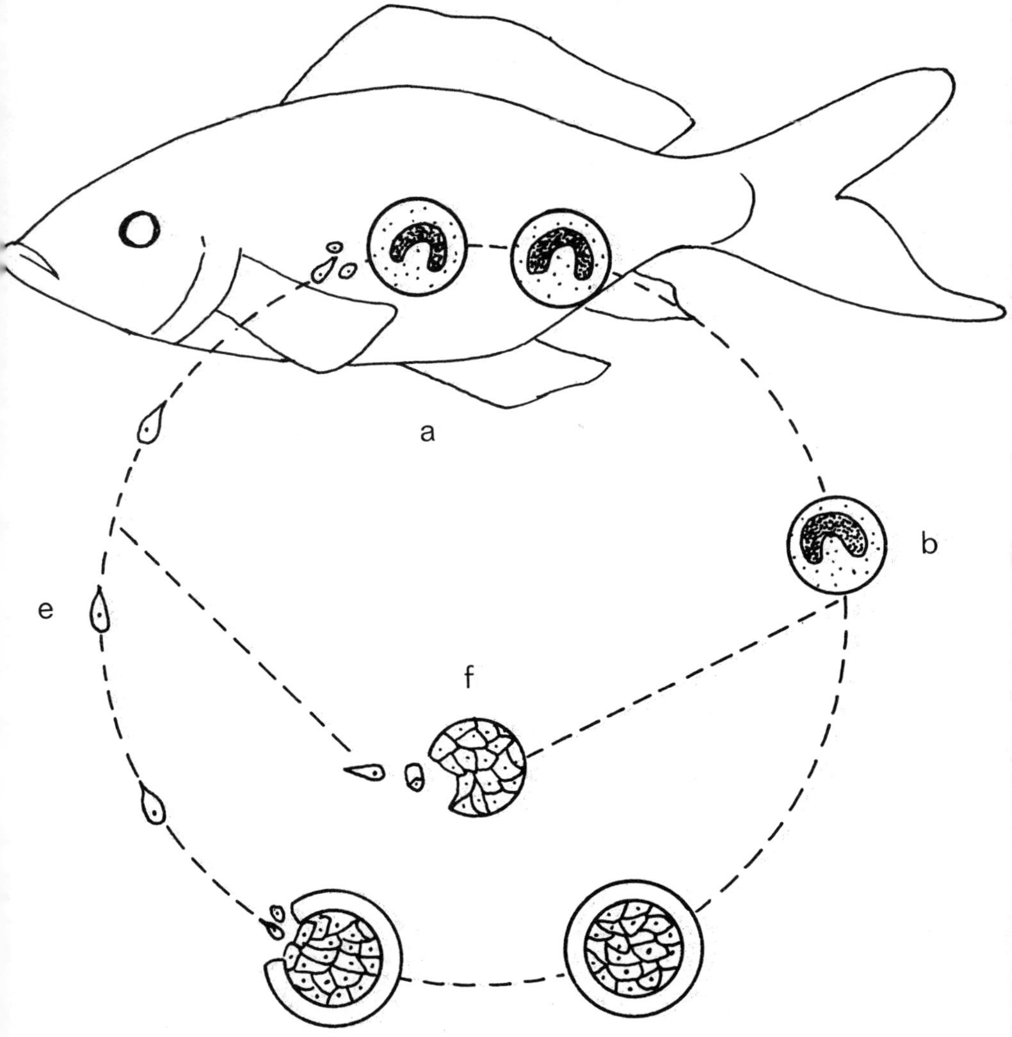

Life cycle of *Ichthyophthirius multifilis*: a, adult cells on fish; b, cells drop to bottom of tank; c, test or capsule forms around cell, which divides to produce swarmers; d, test opens to release infective swarmers; e, swarmers attack host fish; f, if cells forced off host too early, form swarmers directly, without test.

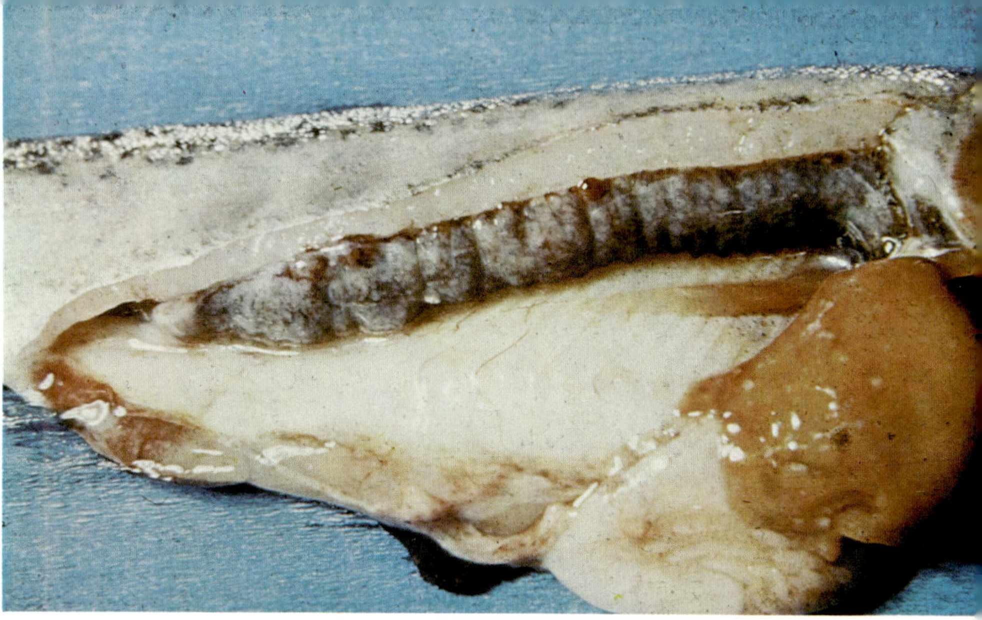

Body cavity of a trout suffering with *Ichthyophonus hoferi*. The kidney (at top of cavity) is discolored and appears pustulose. Photo by Dr. P. Ghittino.

Two cells of *Ichthyophonus hoferi* developing hyphae, a process termed sporulation. Photo by Dr. G. Hoffman.

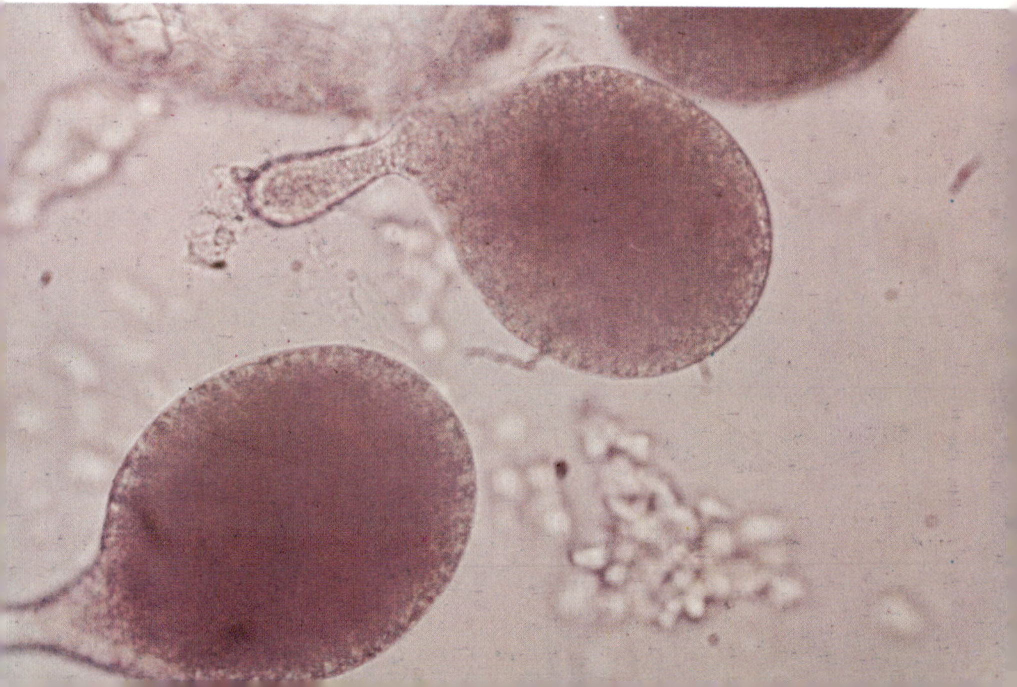

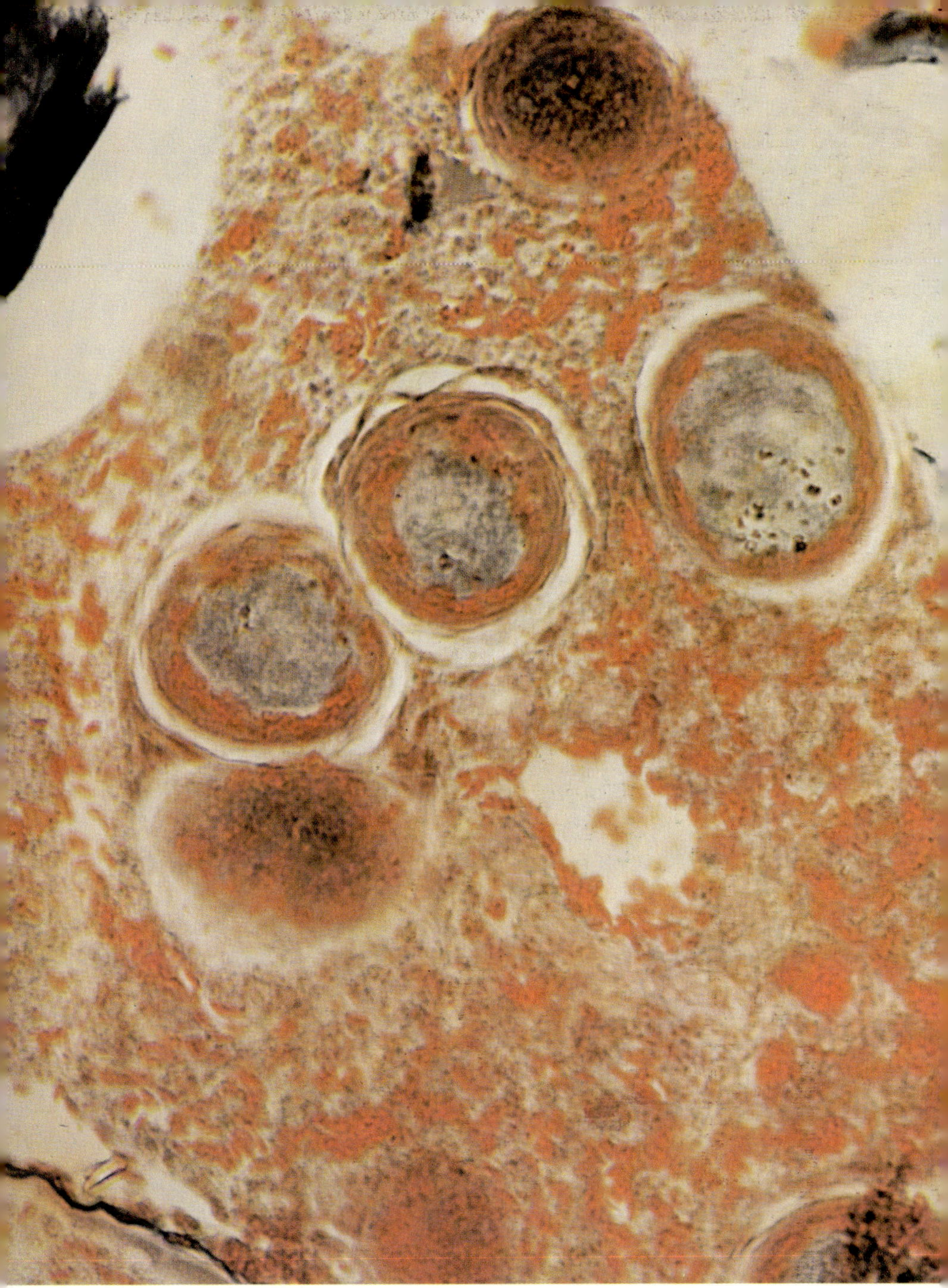

A cross section of the liver of a neon tetra (*Paracheirodon innesi*), showing the cysts of tuberculosis. Photo by Frickhinger.

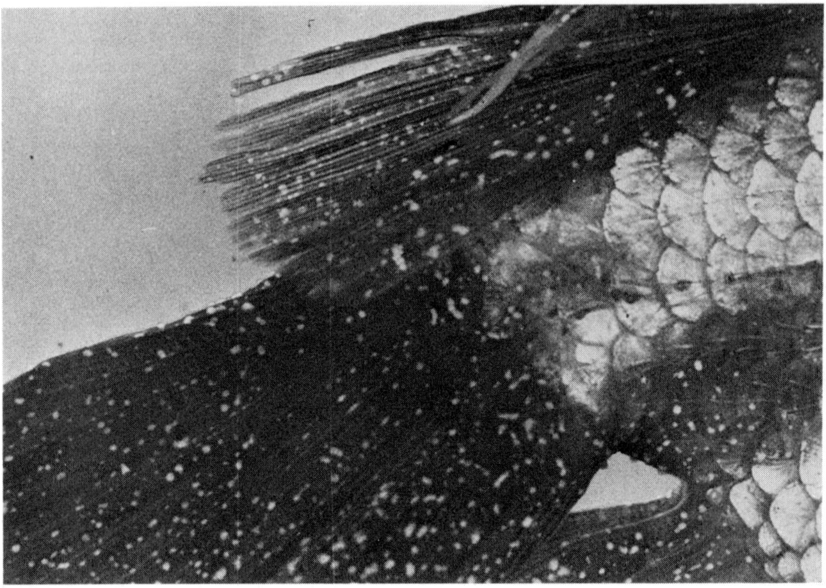

Every aquarist should be able to recognize the characteristic white spots of ich. Photo by the author.

fin, dorsal fin and gills are the favorite sites. The swarmer pierces the skin and may move on inside it. The skin reacts by forming new epithelial tissue which encompasses the parasite. Hence *Ichthyophthirius* lies inside, not on, the skin. Protected in this way, the swarmer grows and reaches maturity. If a parasite is scraped off by the host, or loses its host in some other way, before its development has been completed, it is able, without encapsulation, to divide into a smaller number of swarmers.

One question frequently raised is whether, apart from the forms described above, there are also resistant stages which are able to lie dormant for a long time, unaffected by chemicals, until they suddenly release new swarmers. Could this possibly be the reason for a sudden, unexplained outbreak of *Ichthyophthirius* infection occurring at a time when, to the best of one's knowledge, no infectious material could have been introduced into the tank? Such resistant stages have, in fact, never been found. A more probable explanation for sudden outbreaks of the disease is that a few individual parasites have been living on the fish unnoticed for some time. When for some reason the fish becomes debilitated, the ciliates suddenly begin to multiply in great profusion.

To be able to combat the parasites, it is important that we have some idea about the duration of each individual stage in their development. From the moment of attachment of the swarmers to the moment of detachment of the adult parasites, 4 weeks or more elapse at a temperature of 10° C (50° F). At 27° C (80.6° F) it takes as little as 4 or 5 days. The parasite becomes encapsulated within approximately one hour after detachment. At 27° C, the swarmers are released after about 18–20 hours; at a higher temperature, they may appear after a mere 8–9 hours. A half hour after liberation the swarmers become infective, i.e. ready to attach themselves. They can live without a host for up to 48 hours, but after 55 hours none of them will have survived. Recently it has been observed, however, that under certain conditions the swarmers are able to reproduce sexually. The products of such conjugation are said to pass through a much longer infective stage.

A view under low magnification of ich cells embedded in the fin of an infected fish. Notice that they occur both in the membrane and on the ray. Photo by the author.

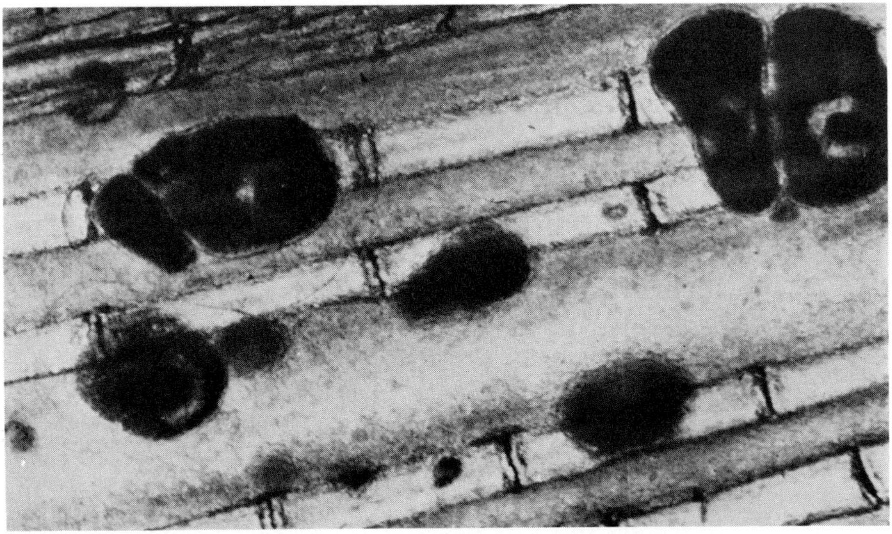

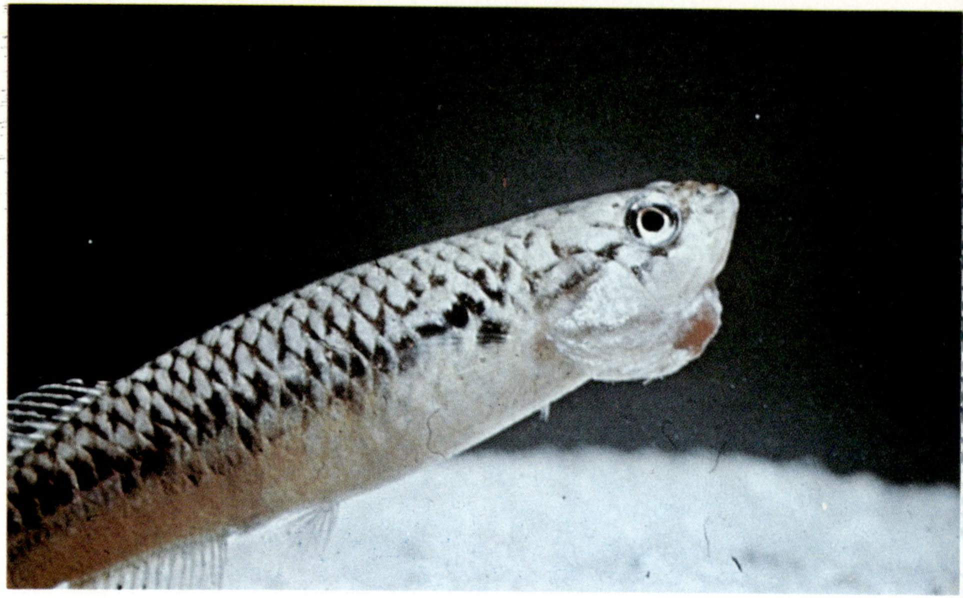

A thyroid tumor is one of the few tumors which will respond to simple treatment. Photo by Dr. Foersch.

Although some tumors and growths may be caused by bacteria and viruses and be harmless, others, such as the one on the snout of this gudgeon, are caused by changes in cell chemistry, producing a condition commonly called cancer. Photo by Dr. M. Thomas.

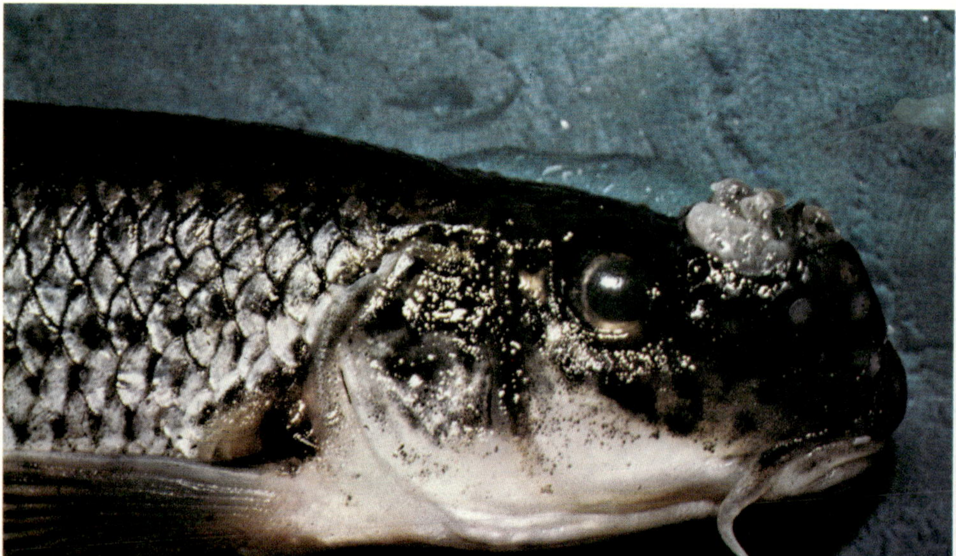

Clinical picture and diagnosis: Infected fish show semolina-like white spots which may form patches if the parasites are very close together. The spots are easily seen with the naked eye, and through a powerful magnifying glass we can observe the rotating movement.

Affected fish hold their fins close to the body and, with violent scraping movements often accomplished by swimming over the bottom in a lateral position, try to rid themselves of the parasites. If their gills, in particular, are severely infested, the fish rapidly grow listless, make no effort to avoid capture, and eventually die. To confirm the diagnosis, it is advisable to examine smears from the skin and gills. Small pieces cut from the fins of a sacrificed animal and examined under the microscope also leave no doubt as to the diagnosis. Where white spot disease is present, the necessary evidence for the diagnosis will be found within several hours after the death of a fish, or sooner.

Incidence and prognosis: The disease is very common indeed and can be contracted by fish of practically every species. An acid environment is, however, less favorable to the development of the swarmers, and at a pH of below 5.5 they cease to grow altogether. Fish kept in acid water are therefore rarely afflicted with Ich. Provided the infection is not too intense, the prognosis is good.

Therapy:

1. *Transfer method.* Every 12 hours the fish are transferred to a tank which is free from parasites. At temperatures below 28°C, the parasites that have dropped to the bottom of a tank during the period the diseased fish was in it cannot have had a chance to produce swarmers. Hence reinfection is impossible and the fish gradually becomes free from parasites. The infected tanks remain unused for 72 hours; during this period all the swarmers will have excysted and died, making the tanks safe for use again. We therefore require 7 tanks, 6 of which will be empty and 1 in use at any one time.

2. *Chemical treatment.* The important thing to realize here is that the drugs are effective only in that they destroy the swarmers; they do not kill the parasites embedded in the skin. Baths of very long duration are therefore necessary to ensure that all the parasites have left the host. To speed up this process, it is recommended to increase the temperature to 33° C (91.4° F) during the day while allowing it to drop to 21° C (69.8° F) during the night, provided the fish

species concerned can tolerate this. The fish should be immersed in this bath for 4 or 5 days, or 7 days if the temperature is 25° C (77° F). Suitable chemicals for this technique are trypaflavine and malachite green. For the past few years pet-shops have been stocking therapeutic agents which are to some extent effective against the parasites embedded in the skin. Infections may continue to occur (special strains of *Ichthyophthirius*?) when even these drugs fail to destroy the parasitic forms under the skin.

3. *Physical control:* If the fish are kept in unplanted aquaria where there is no sand on the bottom and a pump produces a strong water current, the detached parasites cannot continue to develop and the infection ceases after some time. It is important to make sure there are no corners where the water is not moving. This method can only be considered where bigger fish are concerned. Smaller fish would be overcome by the current, which of necessity has to be strong.

SALT WATER ICH, *Cryptocaryon irritans*

Etiology: The ciliate *Cryptocaryon irritans*, found in sea water, closely resembles the freshwater parasite *Ichthyophthirius*. Research into its way of life and mode of reproduction has so far yielded no concrete results.

Clinical picture and diagnosis: Affected fish hold the fins close to the body, scrape themselves against solid objects in the aquarium and are generally very agitated. Usually these up to 2mm-long unicellular organisms are clearly visible to the naked eye. In some cases the skin covering the parasite grows turbid so that the actual intruder remains hidden. As salt water Ich is larger and more easily damaged than *Ichthyophthirius*, this parasite is frequently destroyed during the preparation of a skin smear. If particles with beating cilia are detected, it is extremely likely that they belong to a *Cryptocaryon* specimen that has been torn apart. In undamaged specimens of this parasite, as opposed to *Ichthyophthirius*, a nucleus is very difficult to discern or cannot be discerned at all.

Incidence and prognosis: Infection with *Cryptocaryon* is not uncommon in salt water fishes. *Platax* species in particular are highly susceptible. The disease is more difficult to treat than is *Ichthyophthirius*. It is not unusual for this infection to repeatedly flare up at intervals.

Therapy: Long duration baths in quinine are often, but not always, successful. Long duration baths in copper sulfate are more reliable but have to be administered over a considerable period. When no more parasites can be seen, treatment should be continued for an additional 5 days.

Chilodonella

Etiology: On the dorsal side *Chilodonella* is densely covered with evenly distributed cilia. On the ventral side it has only 8 to 15 rows of cilia, all of which are lateral in position. In the posterior part of the body it has a small indentation, giving the animal a heart-shaped appearance. In the living animal the shape is actually very changeable. The size varies and can be between 40–60 microns. The parasite reproduces by simple transverse fission. It can actively swim short distances and consequently spread to other fish. The risk of infection is greatly increased if the tanks are overstocked. In debilitated fish the disease quickly becomes established and may subsequently spread to healthy animals as well.

A beautifully stained specimen of *Chilodonella cyprini*. Notice the small indentation at the left. Photo by Dr. Lom.

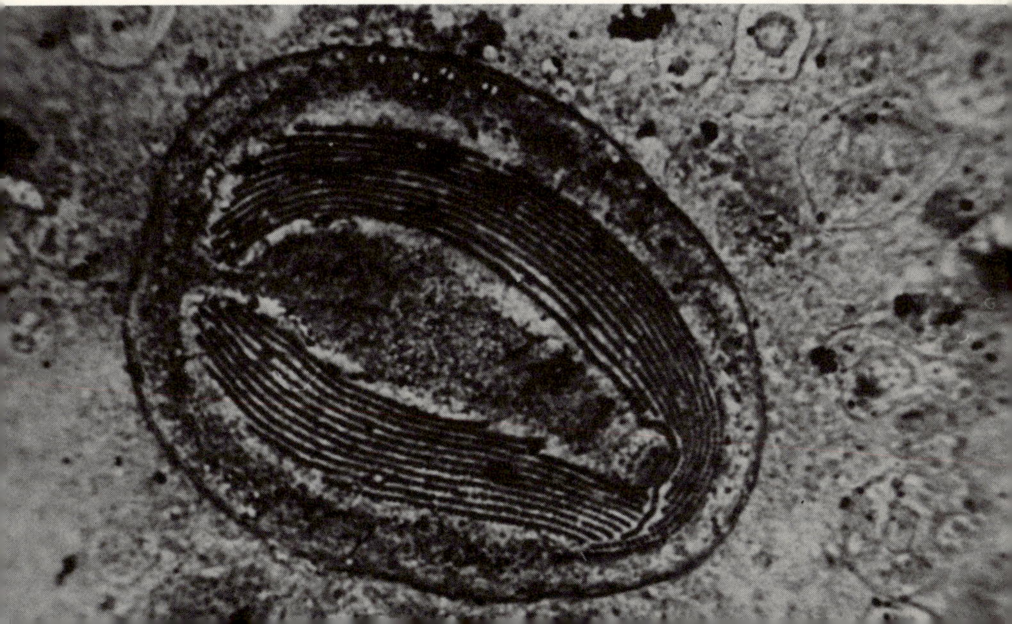

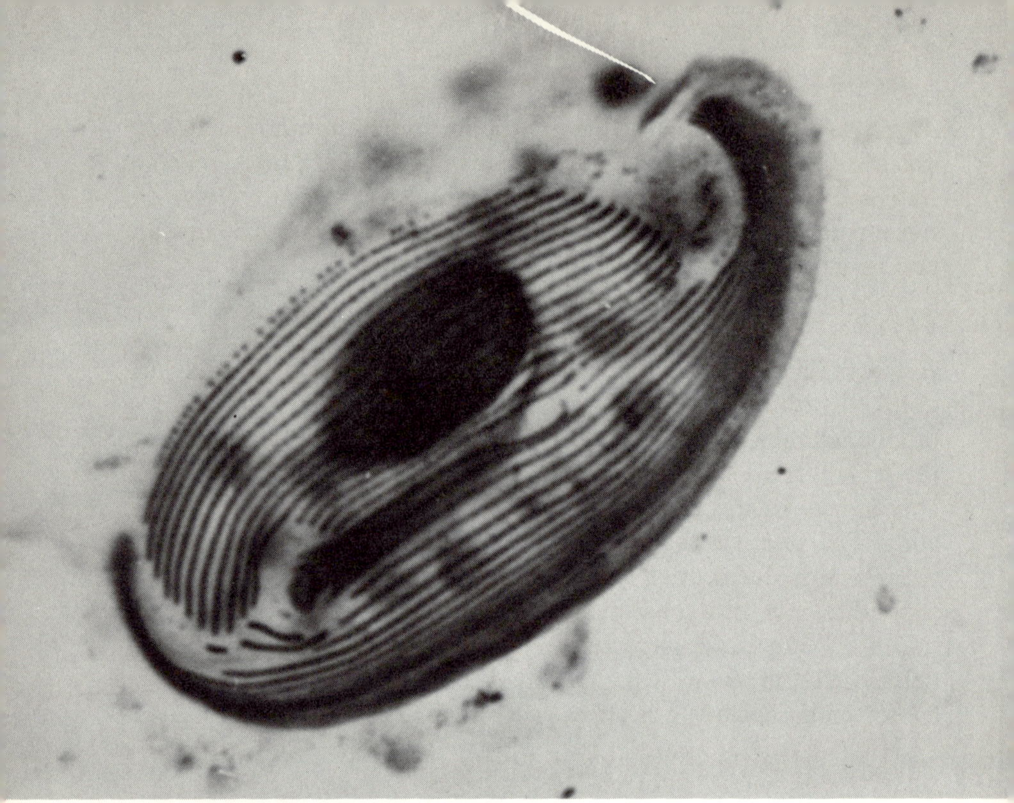

Brooklynella hostilis is very similar to *Chilodonella* but occurs on marine fishes. Photo by Dr. Lom.

Clinical picture and diagnosis: Chilodonella causes bluish-white opaqueness of the skin, affecting above all the area between the head and the dorsal fin. In severe cases the skin is densely covered with parasites and may look considerably swollen. Eventually the skin may fall away in strips. The gills are also attacked and can be totally destroyed so that only the cartilaginous parts of the gill lamellae remain.

The fish make scraping movements and hold their fins close to the body; later they become increasingly listless. If the gills are severely affected, the animals hang limply at the surface and gasp for air. For diagnosis, smears from the skin and gills are examined under the microscope (magnification 100 times). Dead and preserved animals are unsuitable for the examination as the parasite quickly deserts its host once it has died.

Incidence and prognosis: The disease can affect an endless variety of fishes, and in severe attacks the outcome is fatal. If the infection is diagnosed early, the prognosis is a favorable one, but there can be no doubt that *Chilodonella* is the most dangerous of the skin parasites.

Therapy: Long duration baths in trypaflavine (for 10 hours at 28° C (82.4° F)), and in malachite green are effective. Tanks which are standing empty can be considered free from parasites after 3–5 days at a temperature of 28° C.

Trichodina

Etiology: Under the microscope *Trichodina* looks like a fine filigree. This appearance is due to a ring of hooks which vary in number. The living parasite is almost constantly describing a rotary movement and tears off parts of the skin or gills with its hooks. It may also penetrate deep into the host tissue and destroy it. Rarely, *Trichodina* can be found in the urinary bladder. Individual organisms

Trichodina is an actively moving parasite, gliding in a regular fashion over the gills or skin of the host. Photo by F. Leteux, Ozark Fisheries, Inc.

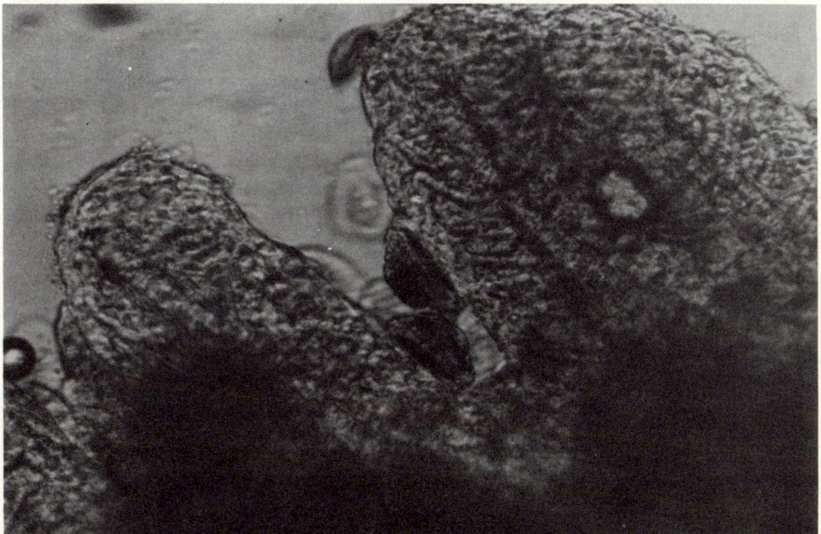

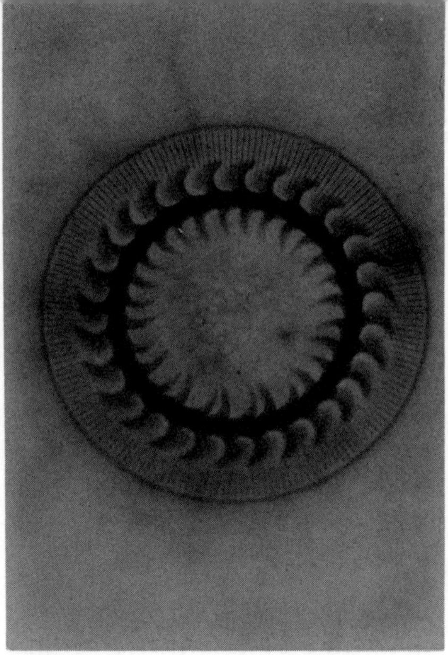

This view of the undersurface or disc of *Trichodina* clearly shows the hooks, modified cilia. In life these appear to rotate rapidly. Photo by Dr. G. Hoffman.

leave the host and attack other fish. There is evidence that, in the absence of a host, *Trichodina* can live free in the water for some time and even find its food there. A number of species have been described, including some living free in the sea.

Clinical picture and diagnosis: The signs of the disease—bluish-white deposits in the skin—resemble those caused by the other skin parasites, except that *Trichodina* usually attacks the gills more severely than the skin. For diagnosis, smears from the skin and gills are examined under the microscope using 100–200 times objectives.

Incidence and prognosis: Individual organisms are harmless. More severe infections can be fatal, particularly in debilitated animals. If treatment is given during the early stages of the disease, the prognosis is good.

Therapy and prophylaxis: Long duration baths (1–2 days) in quinine or trypaflavine are usually successful. Since it is able to lead a planktonic life, it is impossible to prevent *Trichodina* from being introduced into the tank with live food.

Tetrahymena pyriforme

Etiology: Tetrahymena is pear- to pumpkin-shaped. Normally the animal lives free, with a preference for highly polluted water. A few specimens can be found in almost every aquarium. Where they infest fish, they quickly gather and multiply rapidly. Not infrequently they attack fish which have already been seriously weakened by other skin parasites, notably bacteria.

Clinical picture and diagnosis: Infected fish hold the fins close to the body and shimmy. In a skin smear *Tetrahymena* is easily identified since it never occurs singly but, if present at all, always in large numbers.

Incidence and prognosis: Tetrahymena always appears as a secondary parasite, and its presence indicates that the water is very rich in nutrients and badly looked after. Since it affects only fish which have already been weakened by other causes, the prognosis is not good. An infestation with *Tetrahymena* invariably means that the host is already dying.

Therapy: Tetrahymena itself can be controlled with malachite green, but it is important to look for the primary disease.

THE DISCUS PARASITE

Etiology: This parasite, which has been occurring in the intestine of the discus for the past few years, has not as yet been given a scientific name. The organism is an elongate ciliate. One end is rounded off; the other terminates in a pointed thorn and is used by the animal for boring its way into the host tissue.

Clinical picture and diagnosis: The exact damage this parasite is able to cause still remains to be established. Intestinal injuries with inflammation, caused by the sharp thorn, may be assumed. Occasionally the parasite can be detected in freshly deposited feces, but a reliable diagnosis can only be made by examining the intestinal contents of a sacrificed animal.

Incidence: So far the parasite has only been isolated from species of the genus *Symphysodon*. The disease seems to spread slowly from one fish to another.

Therapy: Few tests have been carried out so far. Drugs based on Metronidazol would seem to be effective.

STALKED SKIN PARASITE *(Glossatella)*

On rare occasions a skin smear may contain ciliates with a single crown of cilia on the upper edge. They are attached to the skin by a tapering stalk. The use of malachite green for their control is suggested.

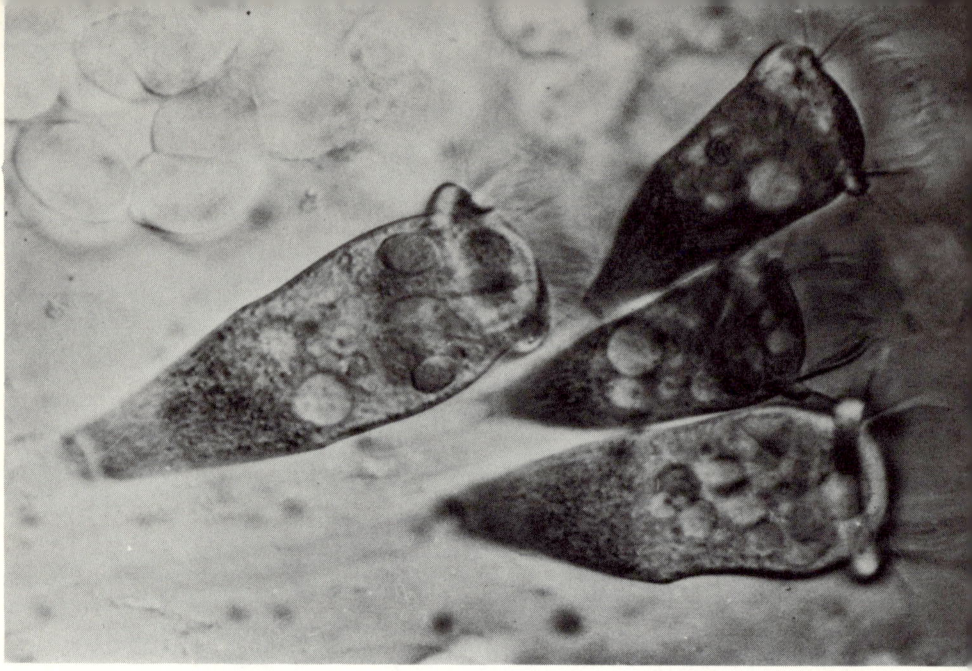

Epistylis is usually considered a commensal rather than a parasite. Under normal conditions it depends on the host for food and transportation but does not do any damage. Photo by Dr. Lom.

Fungi

Fungi are plants without chlorophyll which, as a mass of threads (mycelia), grow on organic matter.

FISH FUNGI (Saprolegniacea)

Etiology: The genera *Saprolegnia* and *Achlya* grow, above all, on decaying organic matter (e.g. remains of food, dead eggs) where they form "meadows" of fine white threads (hyphae). Open wounds on the body of a weakened fish may also be invaded by these fungi.
Clinical picture and diagnosis: The affected areas of the skin are covered with cottonwool-like deposits which collapse when the fish is taken out of the water. Under the microscope one can see thin, transparent threads with darker sporangia.
Incidence and prognosis: Saprolegnia and *Achlya* invade only injured and debilitated animals. Healthy fish do not become infected. The mold is often found in areas where the skin has suffered mechanical injuries, and as a secondary infection following infestation with the

skin parasite *Gyrodactylus* or infections with *Ichthyosporidium* where external lesions are present. The fungus will respond to treatment, but it is important that the primary cause should also be found.

Therapy: Actual fungicides, drugs specifically designed as fungus destroying agents, are too expensive for normal use in the aquarium (Griseofulvin, Moronal) and are not without danger to fish. Suitable preparations may, however, be expected to become available in the future. If the mold is confined to small areas, local application of Rivanol (applied with a brush) will be of help. One has to bear in mind, however, that the fungi usually settle on skin that has already been infected. Control of skin bacteria usually gets rid of the fungi as well.

Ichthyosporidium hoferi (= Ichthyophonus)

The fungus *Ichthyosporidium hoferi* will be known to most aquarists under its old name *Ichthyophonus*. It was once considered the greatest disaster that could befall the aquarium and was held responsible for half the total losses occurring among ornamental fishes. More recent research has shown, however, that *Ichthyosporidium* is fairly rare in the aquarium. In the majority of cases diagnosed

The hypha of *Branchiomyces* and some other parasitic fungi is actually one long cell, as there are no cell walls dividing the growth into smaller cells. Photo by Dr. P. Ghittino.

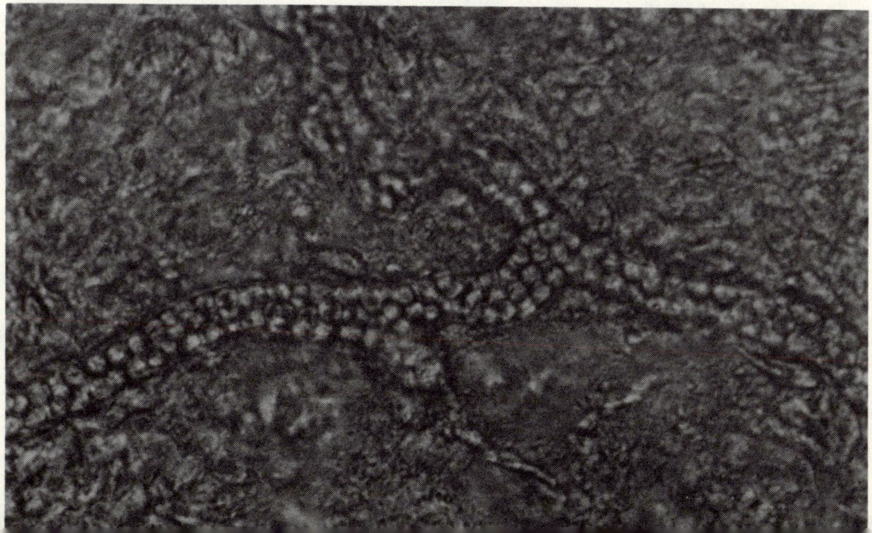

as *"Ichthyophonus,"* the fishes were really suffering from piscine tuberculosis. True *Ichthyosporidium* infections can, however, occur in the salt water aquarium. In fresh water tanks I have so far found unmistakable signs of the disease only in live-bearers and in cichlids. The fungus invades almost all the internal organs. It is found in the liver, kidney, spleen, heart, ovary, the male gonads, the mesentery, brain, eyes, muscles and skin. It forms cysts, more or less spherical in shape, which may be microscopically small but can occasionally attain a size of up to 2 mm. Under the microscope they show a brown color and are less transparent than the surrounding tissue. Characteristically, they have spherical or angular black inclusions. Since very similar cysts also occur in piscine tuberculosis, the two diseases are difficult to differentiate. If squash preparations containing suspected cysts of *Ichthyosporidium*, and perhaps a small amount of added glycerine, are left to stand for a period of 2 to 14 days, the thick or thin hyphae will soon begin to germinate. A cure is not known. All proposed methods of treatment published so far have proved uncertain.

Exophthalmos in fishes can be caused by many factors, ranging from mechanical injuries and water chemistry to piscine tuberculosis. Photo by R. Zukal.

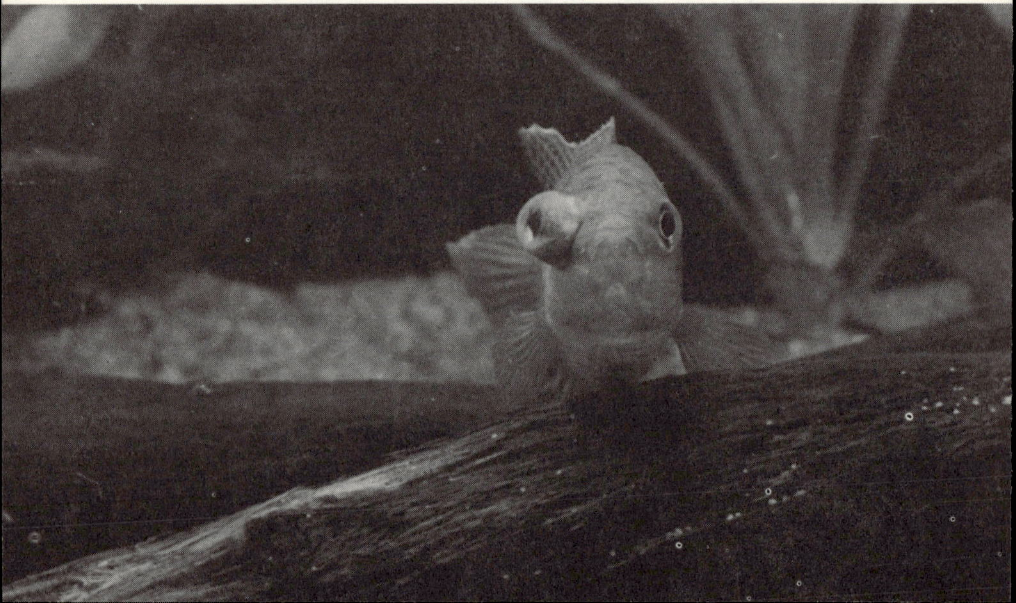

Bacteria and viruses

Bacteria are unicellular organisms without a nucleus that is comparable to that of higher organisms. Owing to their minute size (just a few millimicrons), bacteria can easily spread anywhere. Viruses are still smaller and can only be seen with the aid of an electron microscope. To multiply, they need living cells.

Bacterial and viral diseases can only be diagnosed in specially equipped laboratories. The descriptions below have, therefore, been limited to a few diseases which can be identified fairly reliably without the use of specific equipment.

PISCINE TUBERCULOSIS *(Mycobacterium piscium)*

Etiology: Piscine tuberculosis is caused by species of bacteria belonging to the genus *Mycobacterium*, which also includes the causative agent of tuberculosis in man. The disease is very widespread in aquarium fishes although it is rare in wild fishes. It must be pointed out, however, that the disease is not always fatal. The bacterial foci in the body become encapsulated to form small nodules (Lat. *tuberculum* = nodule). As long as environmental conditions for the fish remain good, there is no danger. But if the host is weakened by unsuitable water conditions, another disease, etc., the nodules can burst, the infection with piscine tuberculosis then becomes acute and can kill the fish.

Among the *Mycobacterium* species occurring in fish there is at least one, possibly two, which can also be pathogenic to man. Accidentally drinking aquarium water should therefore be avoided when siphoning and so should reaching into the aquarium with open or not fully healed wounds. Cuts caused by glass panes from the aquarium should be allowed to bleed freely and then be disinfected.

Clinical picture and diagnosis: The signs of fish tuberculosis are extremely varied. Often the diseased fish show loss of appetite and emaciation (sunken belly, thin "knife-blade" backs). There may also be cases where a fish has clearly died of mycobacterial infection but death was not preceded by external signs. Exophthalmos ("staring eyes") is common but by no means always due to the presence of tubercles behind the eye. With our limited equipment an exact diagnosis is not possible. The nodules in the various organs are easily detected with the microscope. Reliable differentiation from nodules caused by *Ichthyosporidium hoferi* is, however, not possible.

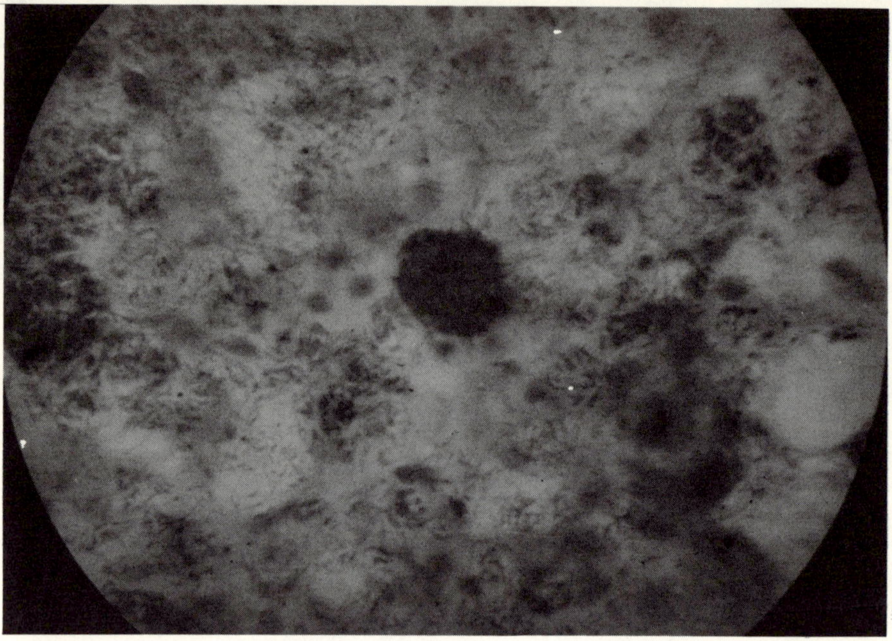

Microscopic view of the bacterium *Mycobacterium* producing tuberculosis in a rasbora. Photo by R. Geisler.

It may be of some help to remember that nodules found in tuberculosis appear yellow-brown, as opposed to the black-brown ones produced by *Ichthyosporidium*. However, since both diseases are incurable as a rule, a differentiation is not particularly important. *Incidence and prognosis:* The disease is extremely common. Fish with marked signs of the disease can rarely be saved.

Therapy and prophylaxis: Chemotherapy is so far not possible. Experiments with drugs used in human medicine (tuberculostatica) are still in their early stages. In practice it is impossible to prevent the fish from becoming infected with *Mycobacterium*. Fish kept under optimal conditions rarely contract tuberculosis. If mortality due to this disease occurs in the aquarium, all suspected fish should be destroyed. For the remainder, the best possible conditions must be created. It is essential to make sure that no dead fish are left lying in the tank. They release masses of bacteria which usually are particularly aggressive (virulent). Dying fish should also be removed.

COLUMNARIS DISEASE

Etiology: This disease is caused by two, for us indistinguishable, species of bacteria: *Chondrococcus columnaris* and *Cytophaga psychrophila* (cold water or peduncle disease).

Clinical picture and diagnosis: The clinical picture of columnaris disease varies greatly. In many live-bearers (although not the guppy) the disease takes the form of "mouth fungus;" white areas from which the finest white threads project appear around, particularly above, the mouth. Such zones can, however, occur on other parts of the body as well. Sometimes the white threads are absent, although the fish is clearly suffering from columnaris infection. With the aid of a microscope the disease is easy to detect. Scrape across the suspected area with a scalpel or lancet to take a smear. If the smear is obtained from a living fish, the wound subsequently needs to be cleaned with Rivanol solution. The smear is covered with a cover slip and examined under the microscope, using at least 400 times objectives. After a few minutes the bacteria leave the tissue and we can see long, very thin threads which fix themselves to the cover slip with one end (never to the object slide). The other end slowly swings to and fro.

Gills infected with columnaris disease, caused by the bacterium *Chondrococcus columnaris*. Photo by Dr. Davis.

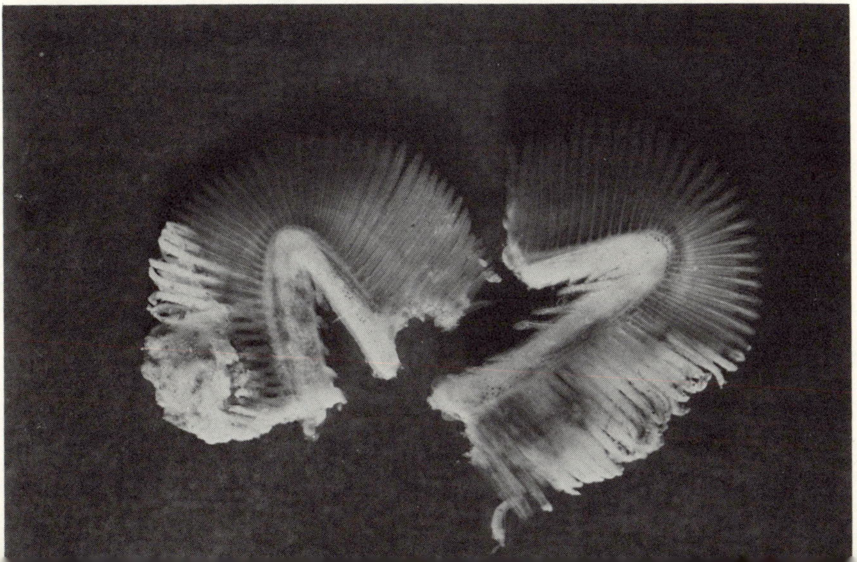

Incidence and prognosis: The disease is very widespread, above all in live-bearers though it seems to occur in practically all fresh water fishes. Whether the clinical picture seen in salt water fishes, which looks identical under the microscope, is in fact caused by the same bacteria still requires confirmation. Once the disease has progressed to the stage where external signs can be clearly seen, the prognosis is poor. But treatment during the early stages is likely to be successful.
Therapy: Antibiotics are sometimes effective. Sulfonamides or preparations based on nitrofuran can be recommended.

BACTERIAL SKIN AND FIN ROT

Etiology: Certain species of bacteria, especially those of the genera *Aeromonas* and *Pseudomonas,* that occur in every body of water can attack the skin of fish. Infections of this type become apparent particularly when the fish are kept in an unsuitable environment, as during shipment.
Clinical picture: The skin is destroyed and the fins become frayed. Frequently there is secondary mycosis or infection with *Tetrahymena.*
Therapy: Antibiotics, sulfonamides and preparations based on Nitrofuran. Above all, however, optimal living conditions are the best preventative.

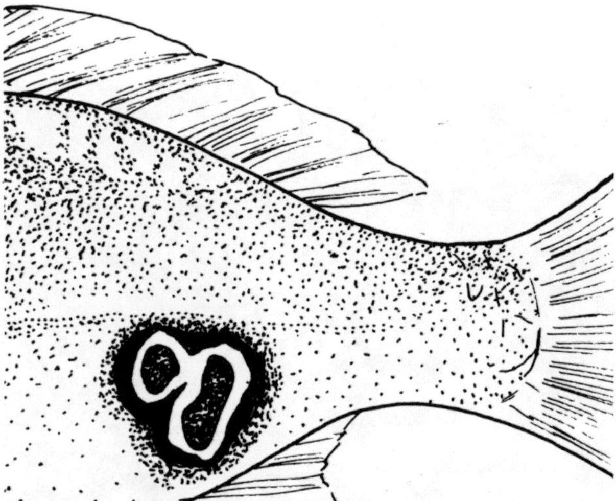

Infections of *Aeromonas* bacteria produce a "rotted" area where the tissue seems to disintegrate.

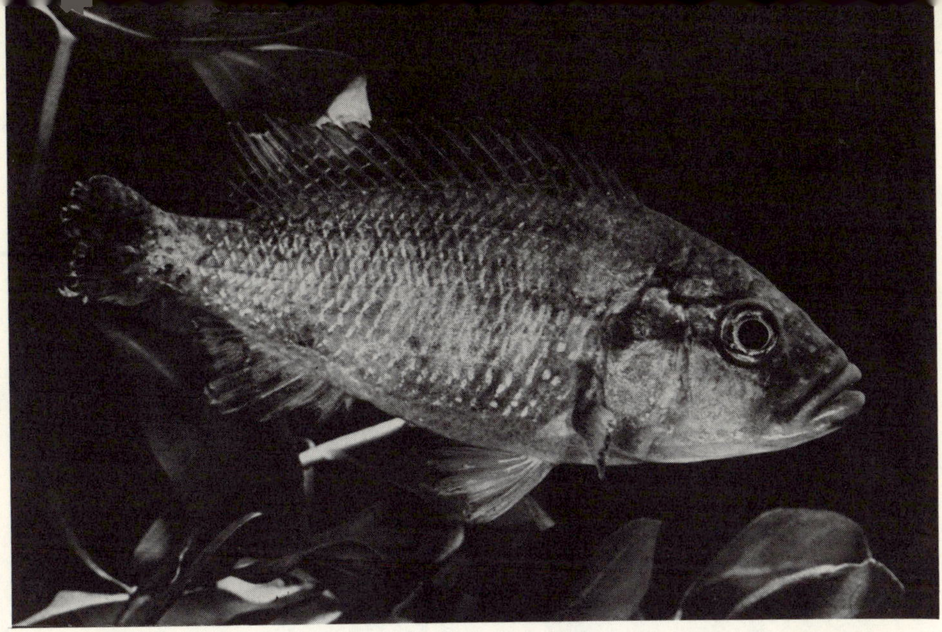

Fin rot, whatever its cause, is usually a sign of dirty water or damaged fins. Usually it is treatable if caught early. Photo by R. Zukal.

INTERNAL BACTERIOSES

Bacterial infections inside the body of the fish cannot be diagnosed by us. One exception, however, is the so-called "false neon tetra disease." As in infections with *Plistophora hyphessobryconis*, opaque white patches appear under the skin. In this case, however, the discoloration is paler. The disease is contracted above all by characins. Milky-white patches appearing under the skin of the cardinal tetra *(Cheirodon axelrodi)* must always be attributed to the "false neon tetra disease" since this particular fish is immune to *Plistophora hyphessobryconis*. Where *Paracheirodon innesi* and other characins are concerned, a squash preparation of the muscle has to be examined for *Plistophora*. Treatment with sulfonamides or drugs based on Nitrofuran is sometimes successful. Often the disease does not respond to any form of treatment.

Viral diseases

So far, little is known about viral diseases in ornamental fishes, and it seems reasonable to suspect that many mysterious losses that occur are due to viruses.

LYMPHOCYSTIS

Fins and body of the infected fish show nodular white growths which look like spawn that has become attached. The disease occurs chiefly in marine aquaria, but occasionally it is also found in fresh water. If only small areas of the fins are affected, these can be removed with sharp scissors. The cuts are painted with Rivanol solution. In some cases, the application of Volon-A Ointment has proved successful. The fins quickly regenerate. *Lymphocystis* infections can sometimes rapidly destroy the whole stock. In other instances the nodules are present but do not multiply, and although they do not go away the fish can grow to a ripe old age.

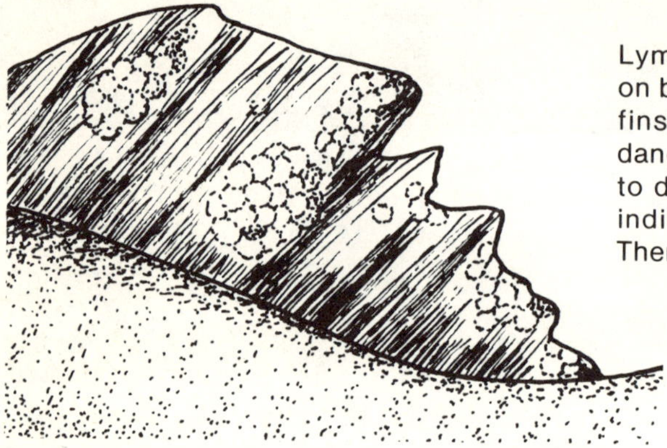

Lymphocystis can occur on both the body and the fins. Whether it is dangerous or not seems to depend on the individual infection. There is no sure cure.

ABDOMINAL DROPSY

The term "abdominal dropsy" denotes a certain clinical picture (the fish have a distended belly), but the cause varies. Abdominal dropsy in the carp is caused by a virus which seems to occur together with a secondary bacterial infection. What is responsible for cases of abdominal dropsy in aquarium fishes can rarely be established. Treatment with antibiotics, sulfonamides or drugs based on Nitrofuran may be tried.

B.—Diseases not caused by parasites

Tumors

Benign and malignant (cancerous) tumors can occur in fishes. What has caused them cannot always be clearly established. If there

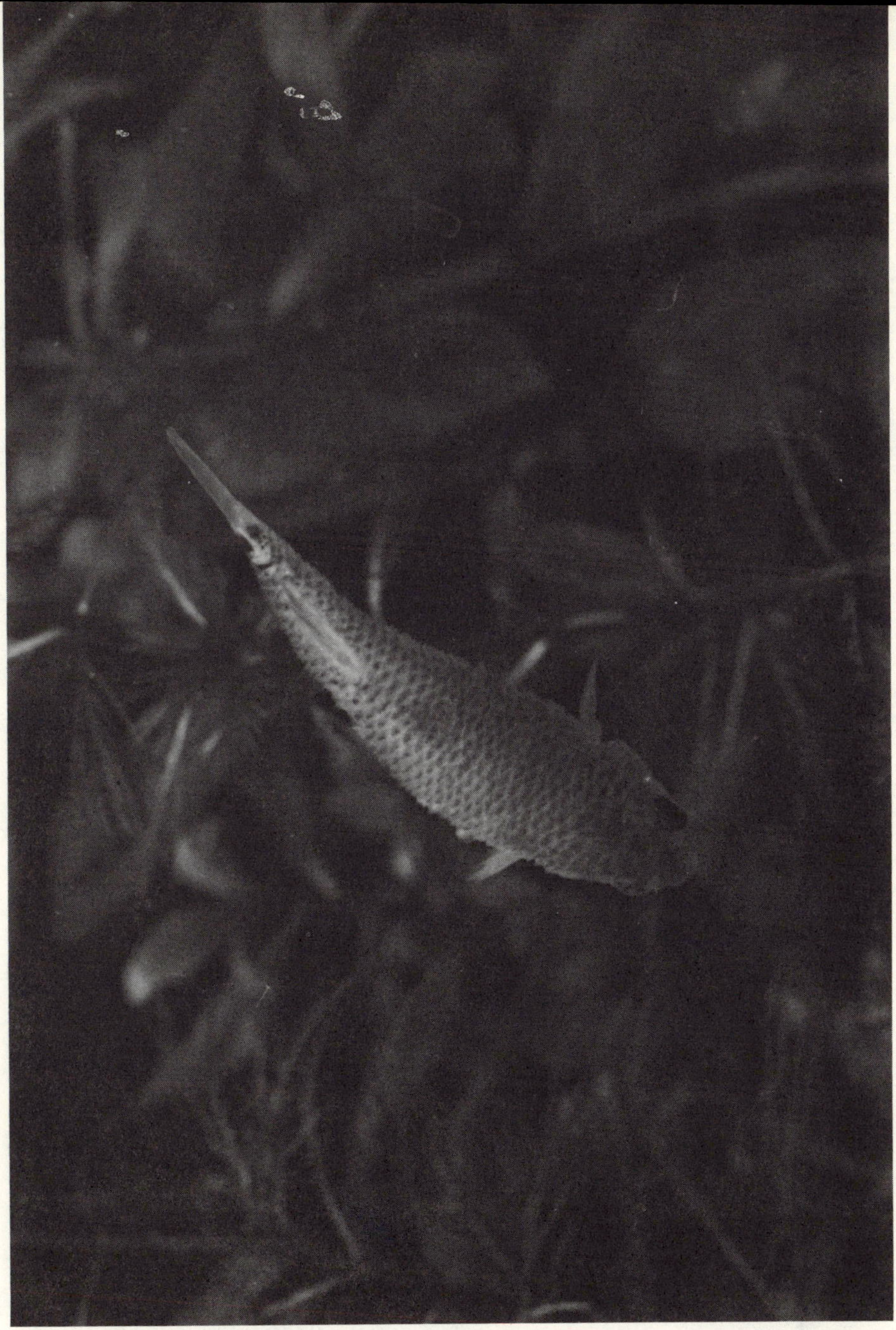

Dropsy may be due to viral or bacterial infections or it may be a response to water chemistry or other improper conditions in the aquarium. Photo by R. Zukal.

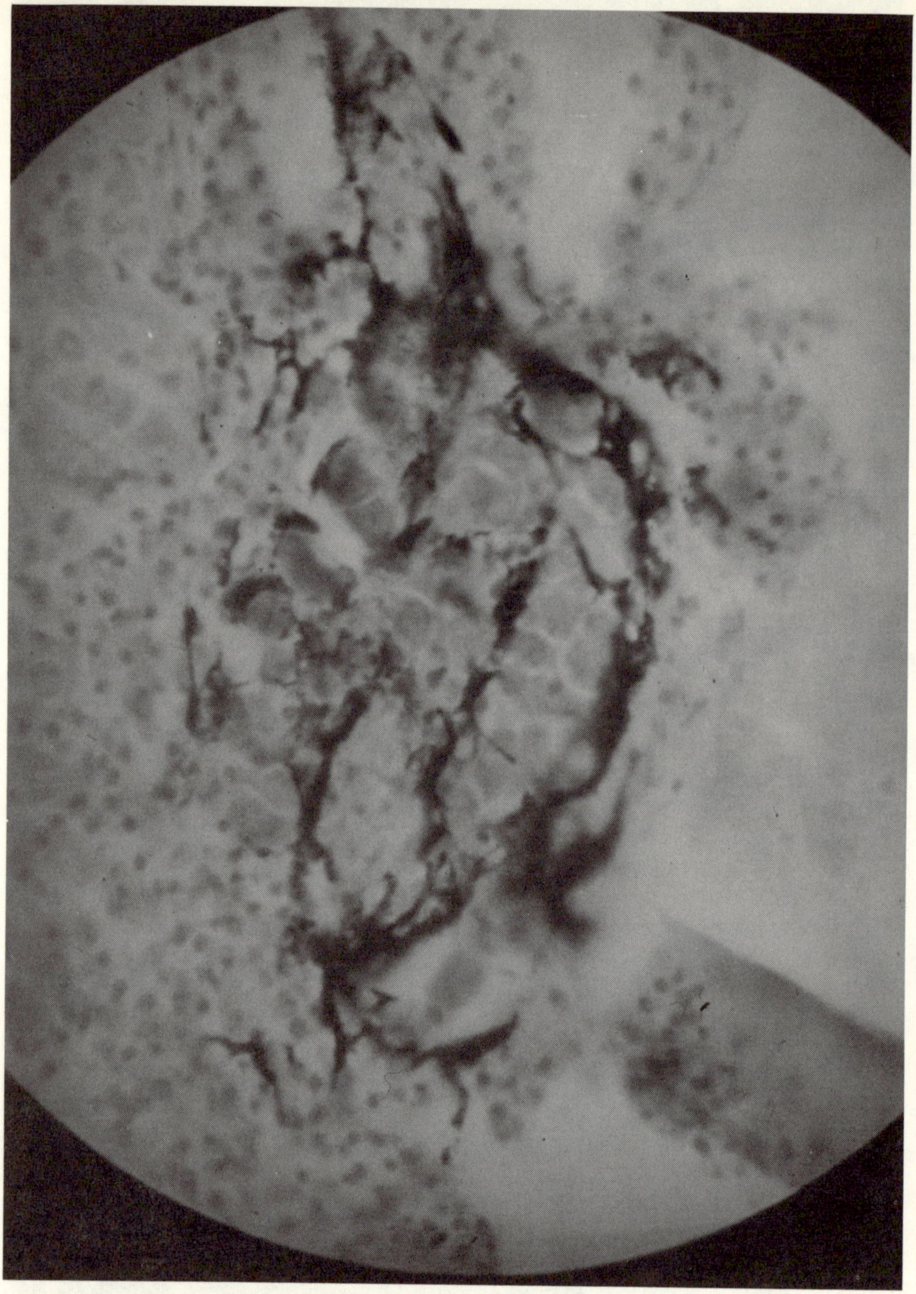

One of the more common tumors, and one of the most dangerous, is the melanosis or black cancer which occurs on many strains of platies and swordtails. The condition is usually fatal and is characterized by black pigment and giant cells. Photo by R. Geisler.

are internal growths leading to distension of the body, subsequent autopsy then reveals the enlargement of an organ. External tumors project from the body like small or large boils. Particularly conspicuous are melanosarcomas. Here the melanophores (black pigment cells of the skin) grow to an enormous size and cause extensive abnormal blackness in the musculature. Melanosarcomas appear principally in hybrids.

One curable abnormal growth is a thyroid tumor. A tumor of the thyroid gland can become so large that the fish is no longer able to close its mouth. The disease may be treated with a long duration bath (if necessary given over a period of several weeks) of potassium iodide solution. It must be pointed out, however, that not every thyroid tumor is curable. If treatment remains unsuccessful, the diseased fish have to be killed, as indeed they must be if suffering from any other kind of tumor.

Lack of oxygen

Oxygen requirements vary greatly from one species of fish to another. In a well aerated tank, lack of oxygen is practically ruled out. However, since only a minute quantity of the air that goes through the tank is actually absorbed by the water (the major part is dissolved on the moving surface), it is important to make sure that the air space above the water is not closed off from the atmosphere (aquarium covers, "built-in" aquaria). If lack of oxygen should occur, it can be rectified by adding several drops of hydrogen peroxide to the water. Secondary lack of oxygen occurs when enough oxygen is dissolved in the water but the fish cannot absorb it in sufficient quantities; this may be due to gill parasites, blood parasites or poisoning (e.g. nitrite).

Acidosis

Cause of the disease: Water which is too acid can cause severe damage. The pH limits are very different from one species of fish to another, but no fish should be exposed to a pH of below 5.5 for any length of time. The danger of a drop in the pH is particularly great in water with a very low degree of hardness.

Clinical picture and diagnosis: The fish shoot through the tank with sudden rapid movements of the fins. Due to gill injuries, they gasp for air and sometimes jump out of the aquarium. Death may occur very rapidly or take a slow course. The fish die in a normal swimming position, often with their colors still at their best. Prolonged, harmful though not fatal, exposure to a water that is too acid results in excessive mucus secretion of the skin, and the skin also shows a milky turbidity and becomes red and inflamed.

As opposed to skin turbidity caused by parasites, these phenomena are not confined to certain areas but appear all over the body. In many cases, a brownish deposit is formed on the gills. The pH of the water must be checked often.

Therapy and prophylaxis: Treat the disease by changing the water. To prevent acidosis, the pH has to be checked at regular intervals. Peat can be dangerous if the water is very soft.

Alkalosis

Cause of the disease: Basic water with a pH of more than 9 also leads to injuries. Strong plant growth in soft water can raise the pH because the plants rob the water of too much carbon dioxide; as a result, calcium bicarbonate, which usually buffers pH fluctuations, is converted into insoluble and hence ineffective calcium carbonate.

Clinical picture and diagnosis: Corroding of the skin and gills. Milky turbidity of the skin.

Therapy and prophylaxis: To treat the disease, change the water. To prevent alkalosis, the pH has to be checked at regular intervals, especially if the water is soft.

Gas bubble disease

Cause of the disease: A fluid (blood, body fluids, water) dissolves more gas under high pressure than under low pressure and more at a lower temperature than at a higher temperature. At a certain temperature and a certain pressure a certain quantity of gas is dissolved. If, for the given conditions, too much gas is dissolved in a liquid, then there is supersaturation. The latter is balanced out at the slightest upset by the release of gas bubbles. Water from the tap (high pressure) running into a glass, for instance, gives off bubbles. In an aquarium which is densely planted or overgrown with algae and exposed to intense sunlight, supersaturation with oxygen can easily occur and soon appear in the tissue fluid and blood of the fish. If there are any subsequent variations or the solar radiation ceases, the oxygen supersaturation in the water falls more rapidly than that in the body of the animal. As a result, fine gas bubbles accumulate inside the animal.

Clinical picture: Bubbles under the skin. Larger fish rustle when taken out of the water.

Therapy and prophylaxis: Transfer to normal water. With filters causing water movement, gas supersaturation can be prevented.

Poisoning

The clinical picture of poisoning varies with the poison. It is, therefore, impossible to give a general description. If sudden fish mortality occurs, the following points should always be checked:

1) Could any paint applied to the tank or fixtures be unsuitable?

2) Could there be cracks or gaps in the paint allowing metals to show through and dissolve? The discus in particular is sensitive to metals, even when they are present in such minute quantities that they barely respond to chemical testing.

3) Has any cement been used without having previously been steeped for at least 3–4 weeks in water that was changed at frequent intervals? If so, the clinical picture is similar to that seen in alkalosis.

4) Could it be that unsuitable tubing, putty, or insulating materials was used? Not all plastics are safe.

5) Might the air pump have sucked in strong cigarette smoke

Abnormalities such as bent backs and pug heads may be genetic or due to water chemistry or disease during the embryonic period.

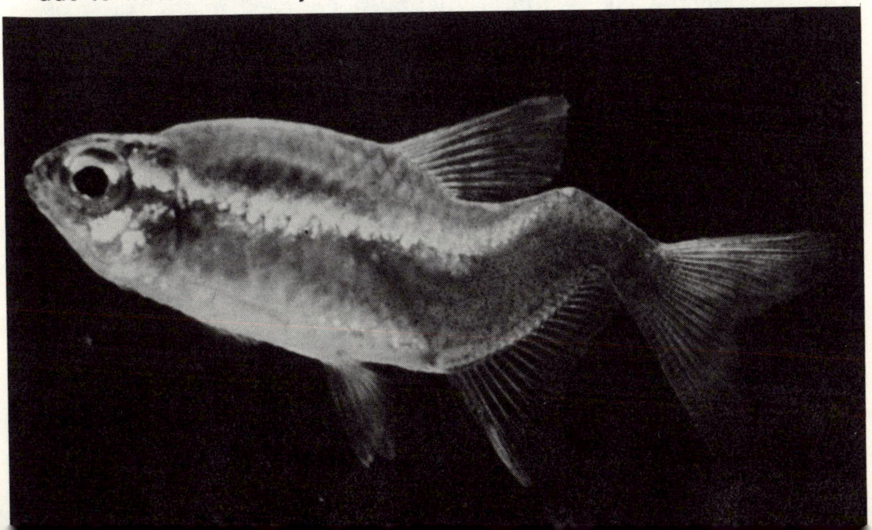

or smoke from a fire place?

6) Were insecticides or herbicides (weed-killers) used in the room? Aerosol deodorants or hairsprays?

7) Was chlorinated tap water used and not allowed to stand for a few days?

8) With regard to nitrogenous compounds, I would like to go a bit more into detail. Protein (food remains, etc.) is broken down by bacteria, and this decomposition first of all results in the production of ammonia. Ammonia is extremely toxic. In the water only part of it is present in the form of free ammonia molecules, the remainder being converted into harmless ammonium ion. The higher the pH, the greater the quantity of free ammonia. At a pH of 6 (i.e., acid water), only the harmless ammonium remains. The clinical picture of ammonia poisoning resembles the signs of acute lack of oxygen. The fish breathes with difficulty and irregularly. If we decrease the pH (by adding sodium biphosphate while constantly checking the pH), the fish can be saved. Once the animals have recovered, it is advisable to change the water. Ammonia poisoning can only occur in alkaline water.

Other bacteria first convert ammonia into nitrite and then into nitrate. Ammonia poisoning is in fact rare. Nitrite already has a toxic effect on fish in relatively low concentrations. If the bacteria which convert nitrite into nitrate are absent, the nitrite content can become high. Reagents to determine the nitrite content are available on the market and should be used at regular intervals to make sure the filters are operating properly. Too high a concentration of nitrite can be counteracted by adding hydrogen peroxide to the water at two-hour intervals. Nitrate only becomes toxic at fairly high concentrations. It can be kept within safe limits by partial water changes carried out at regular intervals.

9) Carbon dioxide poisoning is uncommon. Since carbon dioxide can only gather in harmful concentrations if the water has a low pH, raise the pH to 8 where necessary while keeping a constant check on it.

10) Damage caused by faulty electric heaters does not really come under poisoning as such but should also be mentioned. If one feels a slight tingling sensation when putting one's hands into the water, something has gone wrong, although the fish may not, as yet, show any signs of discomfort.

In all cases described above, the fish should be transferred to safe normal water and the cause removed.

Disturbances connected with feeding

It is impossible, within the scope of this book, to go into the dietary requirements of fish. If a squash preparation from the liver is found to contain many small fat globules, the animal concerned is suffering from fatty degeneration of the liver, which means it has been receiving unsuitable or too much food. During the advanced stages strings of connective tissue can be seen in the liver, though it must be remembered that these may also occur as a result of parasitic infestation. Reddish areas on the intestine, in the absence of parasites, also indicate an unsuitable diet.

A word of warning with regard to *Tubifex* and mosquito larvae from waste waters: they could be poisonous. Larvae of *Chironomus* found in waste waters can cause raised scales.

Mechanical injuries

Injuries due to external causes quickly heal in healthy fish. But if the wounds are fairly large, it is advisable to keep the fish in a long duration bath with Trypaflavine for 2–3 days to prevent infection with fungi or skin parasites. Small wounds are painted with Rivanol.

Drugs

Antibiotics

Antibiotics are specifically effective in the treatment of bacterial diseases. Occasionally they are also recommended for the control of protozoans. Owing to the widespread unchecked application of antibiotics, our aquaria are inhabited by many strains of bacteria which have become resistant to one antibiotic or another. Sometimes the effect of antibiotics is therefore uncertain. The following antibiotics are commonly used in the aquarium:

Chloromycetin = Chloramphenicol, in form of a long duration bath, 50–80 mg/l

Terramycin in form of a long duration bath, 10–20 mg/l

Oxytetracycline in form of a long duration bath, 5–8 mg/l

Note: One liter (=l) is about one quart.

Anaesthetic agents

MS 222 (Sandoz) has proved successful as an anaesthetic agent in fish pathology. Depending on the species and size of fish, a solution of 50–100 mg/l is required (five times this concentration if the fish is to be killed). The right dosage varies from one species to another. New fish anaesthetics with a lesser need for varying the dosage with each species of fish should soon become available on the market.

Concurat

Concurat is the registered tradename of a broad-spectrum anthelminthic containing 2,3,5,6-tetrahydro-6-phenyl-imidazo (2,1,-6) thiazolhydrochloride. For the control of *Capillaria*, the fish should be given chironomid larvae immersed in a solution of 2–4 g/l Concurat until the larvae are beginning to die.

Potassium iodide-iodine

This is used in the form of a long duration bath. 1 g of iodine and 100 g of potassium iodide are dissolved in 1 liter of water. Of this solution, add 0.5 ml per liter of aquarium water.

Potassium permanganate

Used as a short bath for 5–30 minutes at a rate of 1 g to 100 liters. During treatment a careful check has to be kept on the fish, as some fish are sensitive to potassium permanganate.

Copper sulfate

Use for a long duration bath containing 1.5 mg of the blue crystals ($CuSO_4 \cdot 5\,H_2O$) to 4 liters of water or as a standard solution of 1 g to 1 liter. Use 1.5 ccm of standard solution per 1 liter of water.

In freshwater tanks copper sulfate should only be used with the greatest caution. In salt water, copper is quickly precipitated depending on the degree of water impurity. It is, therefore, necessary to repeat half the dosage on the 3rd, 5th and 7th days—more if the sea water is fresh, less if it is older. If you are able to determine the copper concentration, the $CuSO_4 \cdot 5H_2O$ content should be kept at between 0.8 and 1.5 mg/l.

Lindane

Lindane is a highly effective insecticide. It is practically insoluble in water. The fish are placed in a bucket of water and a pinch of Lindane is sprinkled on the surface. The fish remain in this water for 15 minutes while kept under constant observation. If a fish is swimming on its side, it has to be taken out immediately. Rinse the fish thoroughly with aquarium water and put them back into the tank. Caution! Lindane is toxic.

Malachite green

Malachite green is available on the market as a chloride and an oxalate. Usually it is offered in the form of an oxalate which is more toxic for fish but also more effective. Recommended dosage 0.03 mg/l (standard solution 1.5 g per liter, of this 2 ml to 100 liters water). Malachite green is gradually converted into ineffective compounds, so half the original dose has to be added on the 3rd, 5th and 7th days. Malachite green may also be administered at double this dosage.

Metronidazol

Metronidazol (1-β(hydroxyethyl)-2-methyl-5 nitroimidazol) is an active ingredient of various anti-*Trichomonas* agents used in human medicine. These drugs are available in tablet form and can be used in fish pathology, too. Recommended dosage: 4 mg/l (the tablets usually contain 250 mg) for 3–4 days. Metronidazol is quickly removed by filtering over fresh charcoal. In addition it would be advisable to carry out a partial water change.

Nitrofuran derivatives

Certain compounds based on Nitrofuran have a very good bactericidal, and in some cases even fungicidal, effect. Drugs of this type specifically designed for the treatment of fishes may be expected on the market within the next few years.

Rivanol *

100 mg (1 tablet) are dissolved in 100 ml of hot water. After the solution has been allowed to cool, the fish is taken out of the water and the injured area is dabbed with a cotton-wool swab soaked in the solution. If necessary, treatment may be repeated after 48 hours. During treatment the fish must be held in such a way that no Rivanol can run into the gill cavity.

Sulfonamides

As opposed to antibiotics, sulfonamide-resistant strains of bacteria are rarely found in the aquarium. Treatment is carried out with sulfanilamide or sulfathiazol at a concentration of 100 mg/l for 3–4 days. Afterwards the water is filtered over fresh charcoal and partially changed. The sulfonamides mentioned above do not dissolve very well, but the slight water turbidity they may cause is quite harmless.

Trichlorphon

Trichlorphon, 2,2,2,Trichlor-1-hydroxyethyl phosphoric acid-0,0-dimethyl ester is both an insecticide and a broad-spectrum anthelminthic. It is available on the market in concentrations specifically designed for use in fish medicine. The drug is applied in the form of a long duration bath at a concentration of 0.2–0.3 mg/l (active substance), given over a period of 3–4 days. The temperature must not be below 20° C (68° F) and not above 28° C (82.4° F). Trichlorphon is easily removed by filtering the water over fresh charcoal. Where rare species of fish are concerned, it is advisable to carry out preliminary tests to find out whether the fish can tolerate

* 2, ethoxy-6, 9-diamino acridine lactate. Other acridine dyes may also be used.

Trichlorphon. Trichlorphon is effective in fresh and in salt water.

Volon-A Adhesive Ointment

This ointment adheres even under water. If lymphocystic nodules are covered with it, the viruses that have been released are unable to attack new cells. An addition of cortisone and an antibiotic may help to increase the effect. However, the success rate in the control of *Lymphocystis* is not high.

Hydrogen peroxide

To be added to the aquarium water: 0.3–0.5 ml of the 3% standard solution.

The preparation and administration of drugs

Some of the drugs mentioned above can be obtained from a pharmacist without difficulty. Others are available only by prescription, or their purchase entails certain other complications. If we explain our requirements to the pharmacist, preferably when he is not too busy, he should be able to help us.

Where more complex compounds are concerned, the official international abbreviations have been used. The druggist will be able to tell us the tradenames these are marketed under by the various manufacturers. It would be impossible to list all the tradenames here. Some drugs are difficult to obtain as pure substances and are usually marketed in the form of tablets containing additional ingredients and fillers. Here again the pharmacist will be able to tell us whether or not the other ingredients are harmful for our purposes. On request, some druggists will also prepare solutions for us or weigh the required amounts since we are unlikely to possess scales which are accurate enough for quantities of several milligrams. Frequently he may, however, not be able to sell us drugs in such small quantities as are needed by us, since open packets are of no use to him. Perhaps our aquarium societies could help us by buying the more commonly used drugs in "bulk" and passing them on to their members.

Drugs for the control of parasites are meant to kill the pathogenic organisms, so of necessity they have to be toxic. A good drug kills the parasite at concentrations and periods of time which do little, if any, damage to the fish or are at least less damaging than the parasites. The rule, "the more the better," does not apply here and is in fact dangerous. The stated dosage must never be exceeded.

In addition to these drugs, pet-shops also offer a number of preparations. Some of them are excellent. Others, if correctly applied, do no harm. But there are a few about which not even that can be said. It is advisable to check whether or not the manufacturer has stated the ingredients. If he has not, he probably had a good reason, or a bad one. Very likely the preparation consists of nothing but colored water, or the manufacturer was afraid the wicked competitors might copy it. The latter explanation may be understandable, but the aquarist cannot afford to accept it. Preparations for use in human medicine have to bear a label that clearly states the ingredients. In the interest of the aquarists the manufacturers should, therefore, make it a more common procedure to state the composition of their drugs. This would also be the surest way of ousting quack competitors.

All drugs must be carefully dissolved as undissolved remains can cause severe damage. If highly diluted solutions are required and the chemist cannot prepare them for us, we can do it ourselves by diluting the standard solution. For example:

The instructions for a long duration bath in quinine are as follows: 1 g to 100 liters. We want to carry out the treatment in an all-glass tank with a capacity of 10 liters, i.e. we need 0.1 g. For a quantity of 5 g, letter scales are still sufficiently accurate. We prepare a standard solution of 5 g in one liter of water. If 1 liter (= 1000 ml) contains 5 g, then 20 ml contains 0.1 g ($5:1000 = 0.1:x$; $x = \frac{1000 \times 0.1}{5}$). We therefore add 20 ml to 10 liters of water. With the aid of simple arithmetic we can thus adapt the needed dosage to suit our needs (1 mg (milligram) = 0.001 g).

At all times the solutions must be mixed well with the water to prevent the formation of areas with a higher, perhaps harmful, concentration. Long duration baths for the control of skin parasites are given in the tank. During treatment the filter must be switched off or, better, the filter operated only with fresh nylon wool. After treatment carry out a partial water change. Most cures are somewhat unfavorable for the plants, but most plants survive, and it is more important that any germs inside the tank should be destroyed. For short duration baths or quick immersions, the fish is always transferred to a special all-glass tank containing the solution. Beside it we should have another tank ready with water 1 or 2 degrees warmer which has the correct pH and hardness for that particular fish. Should the fish adopt an abnormal swimming position or show signs of great weakness, it is placed in the second tank immediately. In every case it is transferred to the second tank after treatment so that it can be kept under observation for some time. Not all fishes are equally sensitive to certain drugs. It is necessary, therefore, to keep the fish under constant observation when administering short duration baths. Fish in a long duration bath are watched constantly at first, but later it is sufficient to check on them at intervals. If a fish is unable to tolerate a certain drug, we change to a different one.

What to do when unable to make a diagnosis

If this book has not helped us to reach any conclusion because a diagnosis is impossible with the limited equipment and methods available to us or because the disease is not dealt with in the book, we have to turn to an expert for advice. Suitable places to contact include institutes of higher education, fishery authorities, research laboratories concerned with veterinary medicine, etc.

Bearing in mind that a dried up mummy is of no use to anyone, it is best to forward visibly diseased but still living fish for investigation. Many parasites leave the host very shortly after it has died and cannot therefore be detected on the carcass. However, if a dead fish has to be sent, to be of use it must be a freshly killed one. Only when the gills are still bright red is there any possibility of a successful diagnosis. Damp but without water, the fish is put into a plastic bag and stored in the refrigerator (but not in the freezer) until its shipment within at most a couple of hours. Together with another plastic bag which is filled with ice cubes, the bag is then placed inside a styrofoam box and mailed first class or airmail or shipped by express.

Prevention is better than cure

If we offer the right conditions to our fish, making sure they are happy, many diseases will never appear. How to set up an aquarium and how to keep fish is beyond the scope of this book, but it cannot be pointed out too often that it is absolutely essential to know the exact requirements of one's pets if one wants to keep and breed them successfully. A lot of mishaps are caused by the so-called "community tanks" into which everything is indiscriminately thrown that is colorful and does not eat one another. It is impossible to please all fishes! Of course one can set up an aquarium with a variety of South American characins, but such a tank would then be unsuitable for Asian barbs or African cichlids.

Newly acquired fishes must be kept in quarantine for 3–4 weeks. The necessity of this is pointed out in every book. Some experienced aquarists, on the other hand, maintain that it is advantageous to place new arrivals in the same tank as the old stock immediately. They say there are fewer losses this way. Perfectly true, until one day a highly contagious disease slips into the tank and newcomers and old stock alike go to the heaven for fishes.

Quarantine is essential, but it must be done properly. A bare tank with new water is a sure way of killing a fish already weakened by shipping and storage at the pet-shop. A quarantine tank has to contain carefully conditioned water and must offer suitable hiding places and a peaceful atmosphere to the at first frightened fish. Nor must the quarantine tank be too small. It should contain more liters of water per animal, never less, than the tank they will eventually be kept in.

For the sake of hygiene it is imperative that no tanks come into contact with one another. One tank might contain pathogenic organisms which are harmless under the conditions prevailing there but could cause an outbreak of disease in another tank. This means for every tank a separate net, mud lift, etc. Alternatively, all pieces of equipment are placed in disinfectant solution after use. A saturated solution of sodium chloride has proved successful for this purpose. After a half hour at most, any germs that may have been present are destroyed in this solution. Before use, the instruments are rinsed with running water; this method has the advantage of being cheap. In addition, it ensures that no toxic substances are transferred from one tank to another. Not only instruments, but every drop of aquarium water splashing into another tank can bring disaster. Even greater care must be taken when disease has struck in any of the tanks.

What are we to do if an incurable disease is raging in the aquarium? Should we kill every fish in the tank or let nature take its course, hoping for the best? Those who possess only one tank may choose to do the latter. But it must be realized that the cause of the disease will remain even if no more losses occur. Any upset that weakens the fish, however slightly and unnoticeably, might make the disease flare up again. In a room containing a number of other tanks, a postponed decision may well lead to the loss of the entire stock. The possibility of cross-infection can never be ruled out completely. Flies, for instance, do not abide by the rules of hygiene!

Selected reading

Amlacher, E. 1970. *Textbook of Fish Diseases*. T.F.H. Publ., 302 pages.

Goldstein, R. 1971. *Diseases of Aquarium Fishes*. T.F.H. Publ., 126 pages.

Hoffman, G.L. and F.P. Meyer. 1974. *Parasites of Freshwater Fishes*. T.F.H. Publ., 224 pages. Excellent for treatment information.

Reichenbach-Klinke, H.H. 1973. *Fish Pathology*. T.F.H. Publ., 512 pages.

INDEX

Page numbers in **bold** type indicate illustrations